CLINICAL COMPANION FOR

FUNDAMENTALS OF NURSING

JUST THE FACTS

EIGHTH EDITION

VERONICA "RONNIE" PETERSON
BA, RN, BSN, MS

Manager of Clinical Support
University of Wisconsin Medical Foundation

With 106 illustrations

ELSEVIER

ELSEVIER
MOSBY

3251 Riverport Lane
St. Louis, Missouri 63043

CLINICAL COMPANION FOR FUNDAMENTALS OF   ISBN 978-0-323-08526-7
NURSING: JUST THE FACTS, EIGHTH EDITION

Notices

Knowledge and best practice in this field are constantly changing. As new research and experience broaden our understanding, changes in research methods, professional practices, or medical treatment may become necessary.

Practitioners and researchers must always rely on their own experience and knowledge in evaluating and using any information, methods, compounds, or experiments described herein. In using such information or methods they should be mindful of their own safety and the safety of others, including parties for whom they have a professional responsibility.

With respect to any drug or pharmaceutical products identified, readers are advised to check the most current information provided (i) on procedures featured or (ii) by the manufacturer of each product to be administered, to verify the recommended dose or formula, the method and duration of administration, and contraindications. It is the responsibility of practitioners, relying on their own experience and knowledge of their patients, to make diagnoses, to determine dosages and the best treatment for each individual patient, and to take all appropriate safety precautions.

To the fullest extent of the law, neither the Publisher nor the authors, contributors, or editors, assume any liability for any injury and/or damage to persons or property as a matter of products liability, negligence or otherwise, or from any use or operation of any methods, products, instructions, or ideas contained in the material herein.

International Standard Book Number : 978-0-323-08526-7

Senior Content Strategist: Tamara Myers
Content Development Specialist: Melissa J. Rawe, Tina Kaemmerer
Publishing Services Manager: Deborah L. Vogel
Senior Project Manager: Jodi M. Willard; Deepthi Unni
Design Direction: Teresa McBryan

Printed in the United States of America

Last digit is the print number: 9   8   7   6   5   4   3   2

Preface

When I began my first student clinical experience, I felt overwhelmed. There just wasn't time to memorize lab values, metric conversions, or the dozens of other facts I needed to know. So I compiled a small notebook of this information and carried it with me everywhere. Later, as a graduate student pursuing my master's degree, I taught nursing students who were experiencing the same problem.

For them, and for you, I have compiled those hard-to-memorize charts, graphs, numbers, and abbreviations that you must know, even in your first clinical experience. I've added some handy checklists for physical assessment and an assortment of other useful bits of information.

Clinical Companion for Fundamentals of Nursing: Just the Facts, Eighth edition, is designed to be a portable, quick reference for facts and figures, focusing on adult health care. I hope you will find this as handy a resource during your clinical work as I did.

Ronnie Peterson

Contents

4 Basic Nursing Assessments, *81*

5 Documentation, *105*

10 Circulatory System, *207*

11 Respiratory System, *218*

CHAPTER 1

Health Care Terminology

For an in-depth study of health care terminology, consult the following publications:

Chabner, D-E: *Medical terminology: a short course*, ed 6, St Louis, 2012, Mosby.

Mosby: *Mosby's dictionary of medicine, nursing & health professions*, ed 8, St. Louis, 2009, Mosby.

Patton K, Thibodeau G: *Structure and function of the human body*, ed 14, St. Louis, 2012, Mosby.

ABBREVIATIONS*

a before
aa of each
AA Alcoholics Anonymous; ascending aorta
AAA abdominal aortic aneurysm
abd abdomen; abdominal
ABG arterial blood gas
abn abnormal
abp arterial blood pressure
ac before meals
ACTH adrenocorticotropic hormone
ad lib as desired
ADH antidiuretic hormone
ADLs activities of daily living
AIDS acquired immunodeficiency syndrome
AK above the knee
AKA above the knee amputation
ALL acute lymphocytic leukemia
ALS amyotrophic lateral sclerosis
am morning
ama against medical advice
amb ambulatory
AML acute monocytic (myelogenous) leukemia
amp ampicillin; amputation
amt amount
ANS autonomic nervous system
A&O alert and oriented
AODA alcohol and other drug abuse
A&P auscultation and percussion
appy appendectomy
Aq water
ARC AIDS-related complex; American Red Cross
ARDS adult respiratory distress syndrome
ASA aspirin

---

*Standard abbreviations may vary by institution.

ASAP as soon as possible
ASL American Sign Language
AV atrioventricular
AVR aortic valve replacement
A&W alive and well

Ba barium
BAC blood alcohol concentration
BB breakthrough bleeding
BBB blood–brain barrier; bundle-branch block
BBT basal body temperature
BE barium enema
bid twice per day
BK below the knee
BKA below the knee amputation
BL bleeding; baseline; blood loss
BLE both lower extremities
BM bowel movement; body mass; bone marrow
BMR basal metabolic rate
BP blood pressure; bathroom privileges; birth place
BPH benign prostatic hypertrophy
BRBPR bright red blood per rectum
BR bed rest
BRP bathroom privileges
BS blood sugar; bowel sounds; breath sounds
BSA body surface area
BT bleeding time; brain tumor; bladder tumor
BUE both upper extremities
BUN blood urea nitrogen
BV blood volume
BW body weight; birth weight
Bx biopsy

$\bar{c}$ with
C Celsius; calorie
CA cancer

C&A Clinitest and Acetest
CABG coronary artery bypass graft
CAD coronary artery disease
CAT computed axial tomography
cath catheter; catheterization
CBC complete blood count
CBI continuous bladder irrigation
cbr complete bed rest
CBS chronic brain syndrome
CC chief compliant
CCU coronary care unit
CD cadaver donor; cardiac disease
CDC Centers for Disease Control and Prevention
C. diff *Clostridium difficile*
CEA carotid endarterectomy
CF cystic fibrosis; cardiac failure
cg centigram
CHD coronary heart disease; congenital heart disease
CHF congestive heart failure
CHO carbohydrate
CIS carcinoma in situ
cl clear liquid diet
Cl chlorine
CLD chronic liver (lung) disease
cm centimeter; costal margin
cm³ cubic centimeter
CMV cytomegalovirus
CNS central nervous system
c/o complains of
CO carbon monoxide; cardiac output; castor oil
CO₂ carbon dioxide
comp complaint; complication; compound
COPD chronic obstructive pulmonary disease
CP cerebral palsy; closing pressure
CPK creatine phosphokinase
CRD chronic renal disease

CRF chronic renal failure
crit hematocrit
c-sec cesarean section
CS central supply; central service; coronary sinus
C&S culture and sensitivity
CSF cerebrospinal fluid; colony-stimulating factor
CST convulsive shock therapy
CSW certified social worker
CT computed tomography
CV cell volume; central venous
CVA cerebrovascular attack
CVP central venous pressure
CVS cardiovascular system
CXR chest x-ray
cysto cystoscopy

d day
DAT diet as tolerated
dc discontinue
D&C dilatation and curettage
D/C discharge
DDS Doctor of Dental Surgery
DG diagnosis; diastolic gallop
DIC disseminated intravascular coagulation
diff differential blood count
DJD degenerative joint disease
DM diabetes mellitus; diastolic murmur
DNR do not resuscitate
DOA dead on arrival
DOB date of birth
DOD date of death
DOE dyspneic on exertion
DPT diphtheria–pertussis–tetanus
DTR deep tendon reflex
DU duodenal ulcer
DVT deep vein thrombosis

DW distilled water; dry weight
D5W 5% dextrose in water
Dx diagnosis; dextran

EA each
EBL estimated blood loss
EBV Epstein-Barr virus
ECF extracellular fluid
ECG electrocardiogram
ECT electroconvulsive therapy
ED effective dose; emergency department
EDD estimated date of delivery
EEG electroencephalogram
(E)ENT (eye) ear, nose, throat
EL elixir
EMG electromyogram
EN enema
EOM extraocular movement
EP ectopic pregnancy
ER emergency room; ejection rate
ESP extrasensory perception
ESRD end-stage renal disease
EST electroshock therapy
ET endotracheal; etiology; effective temperature
ETOH alcohol

F Fahrenheit; female
FBP femoral blood pressure
FBS fasting blood sugar
f/c/s fever, chills, sweats
FD fatal dose; forceps delivery
FEV forced expiratory volume
FF force fluids; fat free; flat feet; foster father
FFP fresh-frozen plasma
FHR fetal heart rate
fl fluid or full liquid diet
FOB foot of the bed

FP false positive; family practice; frozen plasma
FSH follicle-stimulating hormone
FUO fever of unknown origin
FV fluid volume
fx fracture; family
Fx Hx family history

g gram
GB gallbladder; Guillain-Barré syndrome
GC gonococcus
GH growth hormone
GI gastrointestinal
GP general practitioner
gr grain
grav I, II, III, and so on pregnancy one, two, three, and so on
GT gastrostomy tube
GTH gonadotropic hormone
gtt drops
GTT glucose tolerance test
GU genitourinary
GYN gynecology

h height; high; hormone
HA headache; high anxiety
HAV hepatitis A virus
Hb hemoglobin
HB heart block; hemoglobin; house bound
HBV hepatitis B virus
hCG human chorionic gonadotropin
Hct hematocrit
HD heart disease; Hodgkin disease
HGH human growth hormone
H&H hemoglobin and hematocrit
HIV human immunodeficiency virus
HL hearing loss
HLA human lymphocyte antigen

HO house officer; high oxygen
HOB head of the bed
hr hour
HR heart rate; hospital record
hs at bedtime
HS herpes simplex; house surgeon
HSV herpes simplex virus
HTN hypertension
HVD hypertensive vascular disease
hx history
hypo hypodermic

IC inspiratory capacity; intercostal; intracellular; intracerebral; intracranial
ICP intracranial pressure
ICS intercostal space
ICU intensive care unit
ID infant death; ineffective dose; intradermal
I&D incision and drainage
IDDM insulin-dependent diabetes mellitus
IE immunoelectrophoresis
Ig immunoglobulin
IH infectious hepatitis
IM intramuscular; infectious mononucleosis
IN intranasal
I&O intake and output
IOP intraocular pressure
IP intraperitoneal; interphalangeal
IPPB intermittent positive-pressure breathing
irr irregular
IS in situ; intercostal space; interspace
IT inhalation test; intratracheal tube
ITT insulin tolerance test
IUD intrauterine device
IV intravenous; intravascular
IVP intravenous push
IVPB intravenous piggyback

JEJ jejunum
JRA juvenile rheumatoid arthritis
JV jugular vein (venous)
JVD jugular vein distention
JVP jugular vein pressure (pulse)

K absolute zero; Kelvin
K⁺ potassium
kg kilogram
KJ knee jerk
KUB kidney–ureter–bladder
KVO keep vein open

L liter; left; length; low; lower
LA lactic acid; left arm; left atrial; left atrium
LAD left anterior descending (coronary artery)
LAP left atrial pressure
lat lateral
LBBB left bundle-branch block
LCA left coronary artery
LCH left costal margin
LD lethal dose; left deltoid; living donor
LE lower extremity; left eye
LFD lactose-free diet; least fatal dose
LFT liver function tests
LGH lactogenic hormone
LH luteinizing hormone
LL left leg; left lower; left lung
LLE left lower extremity
LLL left lower lobe
LLQ left lower quadrant
LMP last menstrual period
LOA leave of absence
LOC loss of consciousness; level of consciousness
LOM loss of motion
LP lumbar puncture; low protein
LPN licensed practical nurse

LS lumbar sacral; left side; liver and spleen
LSB left sternal border
LT left; left thigh; long term
LUE left upper extremity
LUL left upper lobe
LUQ left upper quadrant
LV left ventricle; live vaccine
LVH left ventricular hypertrophy

m meter; minim
M male
MA mental age
MAP mean arterial pressure
MD medical doctor; manic depressive; medium dose; muscular dystrophy
ME medical examiner; middle ear
MED minimal effective dose
mEq milliequivalent
mg milligram
Mg magnesium
MG myasthenia gravis
MI myocardial infarction; mitral insufficiency
ml milliliter
ML middle lobe; midline
mm millimeter
MM mucous membrane; malignant melanoma; multiple myeloma
mm³ cubic millimeter
mm Hg millimeters of mercury
mo month
MP mean pressure; menstrual period
MR mental retardation; metabolic rate; mitral reflux
MRI magnetic resonance imaging
MRSA methicillin-resistant *Staphylococcus aureus*
MS multiple sclerosis; mitral stenosis
MSL midsternal line

MSW master's degree in social work
MV mitral valve

N nasal; nerve; normal
Na sodium
NAD no appreciable disease
NAS no added salt; no added sugar
NC no casualty; not cultured
ND no disease; normal delivery
NE no effect; not evaluated
NF normal flow; not found
ng nasogastric
NH nursing home
NI no information; not identified
NIDDM non–insulin-dependent diabetes
  mellitus
NIH National Institutes of Health (Bethesda, MD)
NKDA no known drug allergies
noc night
NPN nonprotein nitrogen
NPO nothing by mouth
NR do not repeat; no response; not readable
NS normal saline; nervous system; no sample; not
  sufficient
NT nasotracheal; not tested
N&V nausea and vomiting

O eye
OB obstetrics
OBS organic brain syndrome
OC office call; on call; oral contraceptive
OD overdose
OH occupational history
OM otitis media
OOB out of bed
OP opening pressure; osmotic pressure
OR operating room

ORIF open reduction with internal fixation
OS left eye; mouth; oral surgery
OT occupational therapy
OTC over the counter

p after; pulse; pupil
PA physician's assistant; pathology; primary anemia; pulmonary artery
PA posteroanterior
PaCO$_2$ partial pressure of carbon dioxide (arterial)
PaO$_2$ partial pressure of oxygen (arterial)
Pap Papanicolaou test (smear)
PAR postanesthesia room
pat paroxysmal atrial tachycardia
pc after meal; platelet count; pulmonic closure
PCA patient-controlled analgesia
PCN penicillin
PCO$_2$ partial pressure of carbon dioxide
PCV packed cell volume
PCWP pulmonary capillary wedge pressure
PD postural drainage; papilla diameter; poorly differentiated
PDR *Physician's Desk Reference*
PE physical examination; pleural effusion; pulmonary emboli
PEEP positive end-expiratory pressure
PEG pneumoencephalogram
PERRLA pupils equal, round, reactive to light, and accommodating
PET positron emission tomography
PG pregnant; prostaglandin
pH hydrogen ion concentration
PI present illness; pulmonary infarction
PID pelvic inflammatory disease
PKU phenylketonuria
pm afternoon

PM postmortem
PMH past medical history
PMS premenstrual syndrome
PN percussion note; pneumonia
PO by mouth; postoperative
PO₂ partial pressure of oxygen
poly many
PP partial pressure; pink puffers (emphysema)
PR per rectum; practical remission; peripheral resistance; pulse rate
PRN as needed
PS per second; physical status; *Pseudomonas*
pt patient; pint
PT physical therapy; parathyroid; pneumothorax
PTT partial thromboplastin time
PUD peptic ulcer disease
PV peripheral vascular; peripheral vein
PVC premature ventricular contraction; pulmonary venous congestion
PVD peripheral vascular disease
PUR postvoid residual

q every; quart
ql as much as desired
qns quantity not sufficient
qs quantity sufficient
QT quiet
QV as much as you like

R right; radiology; rectal; remote; resistance
RA rheumatoid arthritis; renal artery; right arm; right atrium
rad radiation unit; radical; right axis deviation
RAP right atrial pressure
RAS renal artery stenosis
RBBR right bundle-branch block
RBC red blood cell

RCA right coronary artery

RCM right costal margin; red cell mass

RDA recommended daily allowance; right dorsoanterior

RE right eye

REM rapid eye movement

rep repeat

RF rheumatic fever; releasing factor

Rh rhesus factor

RHD rheumatic heart disease

RL right leg (lung)

RLE right lower extremity

RLL right lower lobe

RLQ right lower quadrant

RM radical mastectomy; respiratory movement

RML right middle lobe

RN registered nurse

R/O rule out

ROM range of motion

ROS review of systems

RP refractory period; resting pressure

RPA right pulmonary artery

RR respiratory rate

RRR regular rate and rhythm

RT respiratory therapy; radiation therapy; reaction time

RUA routine urinalysis

RUE right upper extremity

RUL right upper lobe

RUQ right upper quadrant

RV residual volume; respiratory volume

Rx treatment or medications

s without; sacral; single; smooth

SA salicylic acid; sarcoma; surface area

SB sternal border; single breath; stillbirth

SBO small bowel obstruction

SC subcutaneous; semiclosed; sickle cell; sugar coated

SD skin dose; septal defect; standard; standard deviation; sudden death

SF scarlet fever; spinal fluid

SG skin graft; specific gravity

SH serum hepatitis; sex hormone

SI sacroiliac; serum iron

SIDS sudden infant death syndrome

sig let it be labeled

SL under the tongue

SLE systemic lupus erythematosus

SM simple mastectomy; systolic murmur

SN suprasternal notch

SO salpingo-oophorectomy

SOB short of breath; shortness of breath

SOBOE short of breath on exertion

SOS if necessary

S/P status post

sp gr specific gravity

SQ subcutaneous; social quotient; square

sr sedimentation rate; sinus rhythm

ss a half; side to side

ST let it stand; straight; subtotal

STAT immediately

STD sexually transmitted disease

STS serologic test for syphilis

SUD sudden unexplained death

SV severe; stroke volume

SVT supraventricular tachycardia

sx symptom; signs

sz schizophrenia

tsp teaspoon

T temperature; time; tumor;

T$_3$ triiodothyronine

T$_4$ tetraiodothyronine

T&A tonsillectomy and adenoidectomy
TAH total abdominal hysterectomy
TB tuberculosis; total base; total body
TBG thyroxin-binding globulin
TBI total body irradiation
tbsp tablespoon
TBW total body water (weight)
T&C type and crossmatch
TCDB turn, cough, and deep breathe
TD therapy (treatment) discontinued
TE tetanus; tooth extracted
TF total flow; tubular fluid
TG triglycerides
TIA transient ischemic attack
TIBC total iron-binding capacity
tid three times a day
TKO to keep open
TL time lapse; time limited; total lipids
TLC total lung capacity
TM tympanic membrane
TN total negatives; true negative
TNM tumor, nodes, metastasis
TPN total parenteral nutrition
TPR temperature, pulse, respiration
TS test solution; total solids; triple strength
TSA tumor-specific antigen
TSH thyroid-stimulating hormone
TSI triple-sugar iron
tsp teaspoon
TSP total serum protein
TST triple-sugar iron test
TT thrombin time; total thyroxine
TURP transurethral resection of the prostate
tus cough
TV tidal volume; trial visit
TVC total volume capacity

twe tap water enema
Tx treatment

U unknown; upper; urology
UA urinalysis; uric acid
UA/UC urinalysis with cultures
UD urethral discharge
UE upper extremity
UK unknown; urokinase
U/O urine output
URI upper respiratory infection
USP United States Pharmacopeia
ut dict as directed
UTI urinary tract infection
UV ultraviolet; urinary volume

V vein; vision; voice; volume
VA visual acuity
VB viable birth
VC vital capacity; vena cava
VD venereal disease; vapor density
VDH valvular disease/heart
VDRL Venereal Disease Research Laboratory
VF field of vision; ventricular fibrillation
VH vaginal hysterectomy; viral hepatitis
VO verbal order
VP vasopressin; venipuncture; venous pressure
VR vocal resonance; right arm; valve replacement; venous return
VRE vancomycin-resistant *Enterococcus* spp.
VS vital signs; verbal scale
VSD ventricular septal defect
VT tidal volume; ventricular tachycardia
VW vessel wall
VZ varicella-zoster

w watt; week
WB weight bearing; whole blood
WBC white blood cell; white blood cell count
w/c wheelchair
WC ward clerk; white blood cell; whooping cough
WD well developed; well differentiated
WL waiting list; workload
WM white male; whole milk
WNL within normal limits
WR Wassermann reactions
WT weight; white
W/V weight/volume

yr year
yd yard
YF yellow fever
YO year(s) old
ys yellow spot (retina)

ISMP'S List of *Error-Prone Abbreviations, Symbols, and Dose Designations*	
Abbreviations	**Consider Using**
AD, AS, AU	Use "right ear," "left ear," or "each ear"
cc	Use "mL"
DIC	Use "discharge" & "discontinue"
HS	Use "halfstrength" or "bedtime"
hs	Use "bedtime" or "half-strength"

ISMP'S List of *Error-Prone Abbreviations, Symbols, and Dose Designations*—cont'd

Abbreviations	Consider Using
q.d. or QD**	Use "daily"
qhs	Use "nightly"
qn	Use "nightly" or "at bedtime"
q.o.d. or QOD**	Use "every other day"
qld	Use "daily"
q6PM, etc.	Use "6 PM nightly" or "6 PM daily"
SC, SQ, sub q	Use "subcut" or "subcutaneously"
TIW or tiw	Use "3 times weekly"
U or u**	Use "unit"
MgS04	Use magnesium sulfate &
MS, MS04	morphine sulfate
°	Use "hr," "h," or "hour'

**These abbreviations are included on TJC's "minimum list" of dangerous abbreviations, acronyms and symbols that must be included on an organization's "Do Not Use" list, effective January 1,2004. Visit www.jointcommission.org for more information about this TJC requirement.

Permission is granted to reproduce material for internal newsletters or communications with proper attribution. Other reproduction is prohibited without written permission. Unless noted, reports were received through the USP-ISMP Medication Errors Reporting Program (MERP). Report actual and potential medication errors to the MERP via the web at www.ismp.org or by calling 1-800 FAIL-SAF(E). ISMP guarantees confidentiality of infonnation received and respects reporters' wishes as to the level of detail included in publications.

ISMP, Institute for Safe Medication Practices.

PREFIXES

a, an absent
ab away from
ad to or toward
aer air
angio blood vessel
ante before
arteri artery
aud ear

bi two
brady slow

cardi heart
cephal head
cerebro brain
chole gallbladder
chondr cartilage
cirrho yellow
co, con with, together
colo colon
contra opposing
cost rib
cran head
crani skull
cyano blue
cysto liquid-filled urinary bladder

dactyl fingers or toes
de down, from
dent (o) teeth
derma skin
dis away, separate
dys bad, difficult

e without
encephala brain
endo within, inside
enter intestines
epi on, over
erythro red
ex, extra outside of

gastr stomach
glycol sugar

hem blood
hemato blood
hemi one half
hepat liver
hyper above beyond
hypo beneath, below

ileo ileum
ili ilium
inter between
intra or intro within

leuko white
lingu tongue
lip fat
litho stone

macro large
mal bad
mega large
melano black
mesi, meso middle
meta change
micro small
mono one

multi many
my muscle
myel bone marrow
myelo spinal cord

neo new, recent
nephr kidney
neuro nervous system

ophthalm eye
osteo bone
ot ear

par near
para beside, near
per through
peri around
phag eat
phleg vein
pneum lung
polio gray
poly many
post after
pre or pro before

proct rectal
psycho the mind

re back
ren kidney
retro back
rhin nose
rhino nose

semi half
splen spleen
spondyl spinal cord
sub below
super above
supra above

tachy fast
tetra four
tri three

uni one

vascular blood vessel
venous vein

Body Fluids
aqua water
chol(e) bile
dacry(o) tears
galact(o) milk
hem(a) blood
hemat(o) blood
hydro water
lacrima tears
mucus secretions from
    membranes

plasma blood
ptyal(o) saliva
pus liquid
    inflammation
sangui blood
sanguin(o) very
    bloody
serum clear portion of
    blood
urea, uro urine

Body Substances and Chemicals

adip(o) fat
amyl(o) starch
cerumen earwax
collagen connective tissue
ele(o), ole(o) oil
ferrum iron
glyc(o) sugar
hal(o) salt
hyal(o) translucent
lapis stone

lip(o) lipid fat, fatty
lith(o) stone or calculus
mel(i) honey, sugar
natrium sodium
petrous stony hardness
sabum sebaceous gland
sacchar(o) sugar
sal salt

Colors

albus white
chlor(o) green
chrom(o) color
cirrhos orange, yellow
cyan(o) blue
erythr(o) red
leuc(o) white

lutein yellow
melan(o) black
poli(o) gray
rhod(o) red
ruber red
rubor red
xanth(o) yellow

SUFFIXES

ac, al pertaining to
algia pain
ate, ize use, subject

cele protrusion
centesis puncture to remove fluid
cle, cule small
cyte cell

dynia pain

ectomy removal
emesis vomit

emia blood
ent, er, ist person
esis, tion condition

genic origin
gram, graphy written record
graph instrument that records

ia, ism, ity condition
iasis presence of
ible, ile capable
itis inflammation

logy study of

megaly enlargement

ola, ole small
oma tumor
osis, sis abnormal
ostomy opening
ous, tic pertaining to
oxia oxygen

pathy disease
penia deficiency of
pexy, pexis fixation
phagia, phagy eating
phobia fear
plasty surgical shaping
pnea breathing
ptosis prolapse, down

rrhage excessive flow
rrhage, rrhagia suturing
rrhea flow
rrhexis suture

scope examination instrument
scopy examination
stomy surgical opening

tic relating to
tion condition
tome instrument
tomy incision

ule small
ulum small
ulus small
uria urine

SYMBOLS

♀ standing
♀ sitting
o- lying
↑ increasing
↓ decreasing
L left
R right
♀ female
♂ male
ʒ dram
℥ ounce
° degree
′ minute
°C degrees Celsius

°F degrees Fahrenheit
® registered trademark
* birth
⊤ death
Θ normal
× times
= equal to
≈ approximately
ø none or no
→ leading to
@ at
# number
″ seconds
μg microgram

μm micrometer
♀ female
♂ male
+ not definite

∨ systolic blood
    pressure
∧ diastolic blood
    pressure

MEDICAL SPECIALISTS

allergist treats the body's reactions to unusual sensitivity

anesthesiologist provides anesthesia

cardiac surgeon surgically treats conditions and diseases of the heart and chest cavity vessels

cardiologist treats conditions and diseases of the heart and blood vessels

dermatologist treats conditions and diseases of the skin

endocrinologist treats conditions and diseases of the endocrine system

family practitioner treats patients of all ages with medical methods

gastroenterologist treats conditions and diseases of the digestive tract

general practitioner treats patients of all ages with medical methods

geneticist specialist in the study of genetics

gerontologist treats conditions and diseases related to the elderly

gynecologist treats conditions and diseases of the female reproductive system

hematologist treats blood disorders

intensivist monitors and treats people in the intensive care unit

internist treats nonsurgical conditions and diseases in adults and children

medical examiner performs autopsies; analyzes autopsy and pathology evidence related to crimes

neonatologist treats conditions and diseases in newborns, particularly premature births

neurologist treats conditions and diseases of the brain, spinal cord, and nerves

neurosurgeon surgically treats conditions and diseases of the neurologic system

obstetrician treats women during pregnancy and postpartum

oncologist treats tumors (cancers) with surgical and medical methods

ophthalmologist treats conditions and diseases of the eye

orthopedist treats conditions and diseases of the muscles and bones

otolaryngologist treats conditions and diseases of the ears, nose, and throat

pathologist diagnoses conditions and diseases through changes in tissues

pediatrician treats conditions and diseases in children

plastic surgeon treats or restores structural conditions by corrective surgery

podiatrist treats conditions and diseases of the feet

psychiatrist treats mental disorders

pulmonologist medically treats conditions of the respiratory system

radiologist treats conditions and diseases with radiant energy

rheumatologist treats conditions and diseases of the muscles and joints

surgeon treats conditions and diseases with surgical methods

thoracic surgeon surgically treats conditions and diseases of the chest cavity

urologist treats conditions and diseases of the urinary and male reproductive systems

MEDICAL ORGANIZATIONS

AAD American Academy of Dermatology

AAI American Academy of Immunologists

AAN American Academy of Neurology

AANS American Association of Neurological Surgery (Surgeons)

AAO American Association of Ophthalmology (Orthodontists)

AAOG American Association of Obstetricians and Gynecologists

AAOO American Academy of Ophthalmology and Otolaryngology

AAOP American Academy of Oral Pathology

AAOS American Academy of Orthopaedic Surgeons

AAP American Academy of Pediatrics (Periodontology); Association of American Physicians

ACFO American College of Foot Orthopedists

ACFS American College of Foot Surgeons

ADA American Dermatological Association; American Diabetes (Dietetic) Association

AES American Epidemiological Society

AGA American Gastroenterological Association

AGS American Gynecological Society

AHA American Heart (Hospital) Association

ALPOS American Laryngological, Philological, and Otological Society

AMA American Medical Association

AMSUS Association of Military Surgeons of the United States

AMWA American Medical Women's (Writer's) Association

ANA American Neurological Association

AOA American Orthopedic (Osteopathic) Association

APA American Podiatry (Psychiatric) (Psychological) Association

AUA American Urological Association

NURSING SPECIALTIES

AD associate's degree nurse

A/NP adult/nurse practitioner

BS (BSN) bachelor of science (bachelor of science in nursing)

CCRN critical care registered nurse

CDE certified diabetes education

CEN certified emergency nurse

CNE certified nurse education

CNM certified nurse-midwife; clinical nurse manager

CNS clinical nurse specialist

CRNA certified registered nurse anesthetist

DN (ND) doctorate in nursing (nursing doctor)

EdD doctorate of education

FP-NP family practice nurse practitioner

G-NP geriatric nurse practitioner

LPN licensed practical nurse

LVN licensed vocational nurse

MEd master of education

MPH master of public health

MS (MSN) master of science (master of science in nursing)

MSNR master of science in nursing with research

NP nurse practitioner

NP/C nurse practitioner/certified

ONS oncology nurse specialist

PhD doctor of philosophy

PhDc doctor of philosophy, candidate

P-NP pediatric nurse practitioner

RN registered nurse

RNA registered nurse anesthetist
RNC registered nurse certified
TNCC trauma nurse core course

NURSING ORGANIZATIONS

AAACN American Academy of Ambulatory Care Nursing

AACCN American Association of Critical Care Nurses

AACN American Association of Colleges of Nursing

AAHN American Association for the History of Nursing, Inc.

AALNC American Association of Legal Nurse Consultants

AAMN American Assembly for Men in Nursing

AANA American Association of Nurse Anesthetists; American Association of Nurse Attorneys

AANN American Association of Neuroscience Nurses

AANP American Academy of Nurse Practitioners

AAOH American Association of Occupational Health Nurses, Inc.

AAON American Association of Office Nurses

AASPIN American Association of Spinal Cord Injury Nurses

ABNF Association of Black Nursing Faculty, Inc.

ACCH Association for the Care of Children's Health

ACHNE Association of Community Health Nursing Educators

ACHSA American Correctional Health Services Association

ACNM American College of Nurse Midwives

ACPN Advocates for Child Psychiatric Nursing

ACS American Cancer Society

AHA American Heart Association

AHNA American Holistic Nurses Association

ANA American Nurses Association

AN-Aids Association of Nurses in AIDS Care

ANC Army Nurses Corps

ANF American Nurses Foundation

ANNA American Nephrology Nurses' Association

AONE American Organization of Nurse Executives

AORN Association of Operating Room Nurses

APH American Public Health Association

APIC Association for Practitioners in Infection Control

APON Association of Pediatric Oncology Nurses

ARC American Red Cross

ARN Association of Rehabilitation Nurses

ASORN American Society of Ophthalmic Registered Nurses, Inc.

ASPAN American Society of Post Anesthesia Nurses

ASPRSN American Society of Plastic and Reconstructive Surgical Nurses, Inc.

ATDNF Alpha Tau Delta National Fraternity for Professional Nurses

ATS American Thoracic Society

AUAA American Urological Association Allied, Inc.

AWHONN Association of Women's Health, Obstetric, and Neonatal Nurses

CEP Chi Eta Phi Sorority, Inc.

CGEAN Council on Graduate Education for Administration in Nursing

CGFNS Commission on Graduates of Foreign Nursing Schools

CHA Catholic Health Association of the United States

CNA Canadian Nurses' Association

DANA Drug and Alcohol Nursing Association, Inc.

DDNA Developmental Disabilities Nurses Association

DNA Dermatology Nurses Association

ENA Emergency Nurses Association

FNIF Florence Nightingale International Foundation

FNS Frontier Nursing Service

ICLRN Interagency Council on Library Resources for Nursing

INS Intravenous Nurses Society

NADNA National Association of Directors of Nursing in Long-Term Care

NAHC National Association of Home Care

NAHCR National Association for Health Care Recruitment

NAHN National Association of Hispanic Nurses

NANDA- I NANDA International (formerly the North American Nursing Diagnosis Association)

NANN National Association of Neonatal Nurses

NANP National Alliance of Nurse Practitioners

NANPRH National Association of Nurse Practitioners in Reproductive Health

NAON National Association of Orthopaedic Nurses, Inc.

NAPN National Association of Physician Nurses

NAPNAP National Association of Pediatric Nurse Associates and Practitioners

NAPNES National Association for Practical Nurse Education and Service

NASN National Association of School Nurses

NBNA National Black Nurses Association, Inc.

NCCDN National Consortium of Chemical Dependency Nurses

NCF Nurses Christian Fellowship
NCSBON National Council of State Boards of Nursing, Inc.
NEF Nurses Educational Funds, Inc.
NEHW Nurses Environmental Health Watch
NFLPN National Federation of Licensed Practical Nurses, Inc.
NFNA National Flight Nurses Association
NFSNO National Federation of Specialty Nursing Organizations
NGNA National Gerontological Nursing Association
NHPA Nurse Healers Professional Associates
NLN National League for Nursing
NMCHC National Maternal and Child Health Clearinghouse
NNBA National Nurses in Business Association
NNSA National Nurses Society on Addictions
NNSDO National Nursing Staff Development Organization
NOADN National Organization for Associate Degree Nurses
NONPF National Organization of Nurse Practitioner Faculties
NOVA Nurse Organization of Veterans Affairs
NOWWN National Organization of World War Nurses
NSNA National Student Nurses' Association
ONS Oncology Nursing Society
RANCA Retired Army Nurse Corps Association
RNS Respiratory Nursing Society
SERPMHN Society for Education and Research in Psychiatric Mental Health Nursing
SGNA Society of Gastroenterology Nurses and Associates, Inc.

SOHEN Society of Otorhinolaryngology and Head/
   Neck Nurses
SPN Society of Pediatric Nurses
SRAFN Society of Retired Air Force Nurses, Inc.
SRS Society of Rogerian Scholars
SVN Society for Vascular Nursing
TNS Transcultural Nursing Society
VNAA Visiting Nurse Association of America

BODY REGIONS

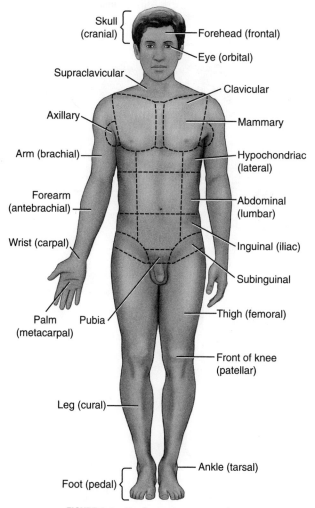

FIGURE 1-1 Body regions: anterior.

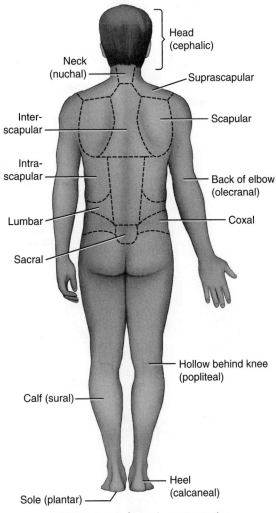

FIGURE 1-2 Body regions: posterior.

BODY CAVITIES

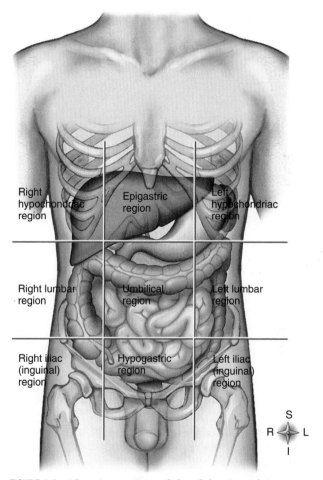

FIGURE 1-3   The nine regions of the abdominopelvic cavity. (From Patton K, Thibodeau G: *Structure and function of the human body*, ed 14, St. Louis, 2012, Mosby.)

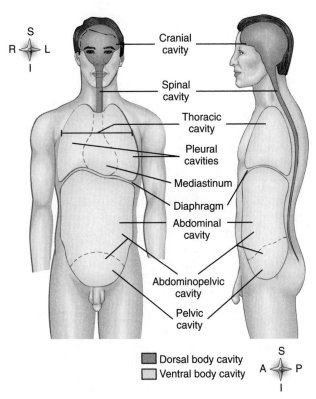

FIGURE 1-4 Body cavities. (From Patton K, Thibodeau G: *Structure and function of the human body*, ed 14, St. Louis, 2012, Mosby.)

DIRECTIONS AND PLANES

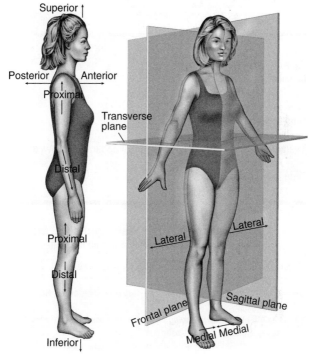

FIGURE 1-5 Directions and planes of the body. (From Patton K, Thibodeau G: *Structure and function of the human body*, ed 14, St. Louis, 2012, Mosby.)

CHAPTER 2

Medications: Calculations and Administration

For an in-depth study of medications, calculations, and administration, consult the following publications

Clayton BC, Stock YN: *Basic pharmacology for nurses*, ed 15, St. Louis, 2010, Mosby.

Skidmore-Roth L: *Mosby's 2012 nursing drug reference*, ed 25, St. Louis, 2012, Mosby.

Workman ML et al: *Understanding pharmacology: essentials for medication safety*, St. Louis, 2011, Mosby.

EQUIVALENT MEASURES
Metric System
To change from a larger to a smaller unit, MULTIPLY the number by 10, 100, and so on or move the decimal point to the RIGHT. To change from a smaller to larger unit, DIVIDE the number by 10, 100, and so on or move the decimal to the LEFT.

Weight

1 kilogram (kg/Kg) = 1000 grams (gm)

1 gram (Gm/gm/g/G) = 1000 milligrams (mg)

1 milligram (mg) = 1000 micrograms (mcg)

Volume

1 liter (L) = 1000 milliliters (mL)

1 deciliter (dL) = 100 milliliters (mL)

1 milliliter (mL) = 1 cubic centimeter (cc)

Length

1 meter (m) = 100 centimeters (cm)

1 meter (m) = 1000 millimeters (mm)

1 centimeter (cm) = 10 millimeters (mm)

Apothecary System

Weight: grains (gr); volume: minims (m), drams (dr), ounces (oz)

Metric-to-Apothecary Conversions

Grams to grains: Multiply grams (gm) by 15

Milligrams to grains: Divide milligrams (mg) by 60

Apothecary-to-Metric Conversions

Grains to grams: Divide grains (gr) by 15

Grains to milligrams: Multiply grains (gr) by 60

Household System
Weight

1 tablespoon (tbsp/T) = 3 teaspoons (tsp/t)

1 cup (c) = 16 tablespoons (tbsp/T)

1 pound (lb) = 16 ounces (oz)

Volume

1 gallon (gal) = 4 quarts (qt)

1 quart (qt) = 2 pints (pt)

1 pint (pt) = 2 cups (c)

1 cup (c) = 8 ounces (oz)

30 cc = 1 ounce (oz)

Kilogram-to-Pound Conversions

Kilograms to pounds: Multiply kilograms (kg) by 2.2

Pounds to kilograms: Divide pounds (lb) by 2.2

Household-Metric Conversions

15 drops (gtt) = 1 mL

1 tsp/t = 5 mL

1 tbsp/T = 15 mL

1 cup/c = 240 mL

1 pint/pt = ≈480 mL

1 quart/qt = ≈960 mL

1 gallon/gal = ≈3785 mL or 4 L

CALCULATIONS
Calculating Strength of a Solution
Solution strength: Desired solution:

$$\frac{X}{100} = \frac{\text{Amount of drug desired}}{\text{Amount of finished solution}}$$

Pediatric Calculations

$$\text{Child's dose} = \frac{\text{Child's body surface area (BSA)}}{1.7}$$

Calculating IV Drip Rates
The *drops per 1 ml* is the number of drops needed to fill a 1-mL syringe.

The *rate* is the number of milliliters per hour.

The *drip rate* is the amount of volume divided by the time needed to infuse.

Following is the equation that can be used to calculate IV drip rates:

$$\frac{\text{Total volume}}{\text{Total time}} = \frac{\text{mL}}{1\text{ minute}} \times \frac{\text{No. of gtt}}{\text{mL}} = \frac{\text{Drops}}{\text{Minute}}$$

Microdrops: A Simple Calculation

   10 drops or gtt: mL/hr = gtt/min per micro
      divided by 6

   15 drops or gtt: mL/hr = gtt/min per micro
      divided by 4

   20 drops or gtt: mL/hr = gtt/min per micro
      divided by 3

60 drops or gtt/mL: mL/hr = gtt/min

COMMON DRUG TERMINOLOGY
General

Absorption The passage of drug molecules into the blood

Abuse A maladaptive pattern of drug usage

Allergic reaction An unpredictable response to a drug

Biotransformation Drug metabolism from an active to an inactive state

Classification Indicates the effect on a body system

Distribution How a drug is absorbed into the body tissues

Duration Length of time in the body

Excretion The exit of the drug from the body

Form Determines the routes of administration

Genetic difference The makeup by which a person's genetic background may affect a drug's actions in the body

Half-life Time of elimination from body

Idiosyncratic Drugs that are overactive or underactive

Interactions When one drug modifies the actions of another

Medication A substance used in the treatment, cure, relief, or prevention of disease

Onset First response of drug in the body

Peak Highest level of drug in the body

Pharmacokinetics The study of how drugs enter the body, reach their site of action, are metabolized, and exit the body

Physiologic variables The normal difference between men and women and differences in weight may affect the metabolism of a drug

Plateau Concentration of scheduled doses

Side effects Unintended secondary effects

Standards Guidelines for purity and quality of a drug
Therapeutic Beneficial level of drug
Tolerance Low response to a drug
Toxic Not beneficial or lethal level of drug
Trough Lowest level of drug in the body

Drug Dependence

A person may be considered dependent on a drug if he or she possesses at least three of the following qualities over a 12-month period:
- Consumes larger doses than intended
- Consumes drug for a longer time period than intended
- Frequent intoxication
- Withdrawal symptoms when away from substance
- Work or social activities are given up to consume more substance
- Continues to use substance despite information or warnings of harm
- Increased time is spent acquiring substances
- Marked tolerance for substance

Modified from American Psychiatric Association: *Diagnostic and statistical manual of mental disorders (DSM-IV)*, rev ed 4, Washington, DC, 2004.

Controlled Substances
Schedule I Highest potential for abuse: heroin, LSD, marijuana
Schedule II High potential for abuse: opioids amphetamines, barbiturates
Schedule III Potential for abuse: steroids, codeine, ketamine, hydrocodone

Schedule IV Low potential for abuse: Valium, Xanax, phenobarbital

Schedule V Lowest potential for abuse: cough suppressants

Routes of Administration with Abbreviations

Oral (PO), sublingual (SL), buccal (B), rectal (PR), topical (T), subcutaneous (SC or SQ), intradermal (ID), intramuscular (IM), intravenous (IV), inhalation (IH), transdermal patch (TD), intrathecal (IT), intraosseous (IO), intraperitoneal (IP), intrapleural (IPL), and intraarterial (IA)

Types of Drug Preparations

Aerosol spray, capsule (coated), cream (nongreasy), elixir (alcohol), extract (concentrated), gel (clear, semisolid), liniment (oily), lotion, lozenge, ointment (semisolid), paste (thicker than ointment), pills, powder (ground drug), spirit (alcohol), suppository (dissolves at body temperature), syrup (sugar based), tablet (coated), tincture (diluted alcohol), transdermal (absorbed)

Therapeutic Drugs

Palliative Gives relief; example: pain medications

Curative Cures disease; example: antibiotics

Supportive Helps body's functions; example: blood pressure medications

Destructive Destroys cells; example: chemotherapy

Restorative Returns to health; example: vitamins

Common Allergic Responses

Difficulty breathing, palpitations, skin rashes, nausea, vomiting, pruritus, rhinitis, tearing, wheezing, diarrhea. *Report all allergic responses.*

DRUG SAFETY
Ten Patient Rights
1. Right patient
2. Right drug
3. Right dose
4. Right route
5. Right time
6. Right assessment
7. Right documentation
8. Right to know
9. Right evaluation
10. Right to refuse

Six Rights for Safe Medication Administration
1. The right to a complete written order
2. The right to a correct dispensed medication
3. The right to have access to drug and patient information
4. The right to have policies on medication administration
5. The right to identify problems in the system
6. The right to stop, think, and be vigilant about medication administration

---

Adapted from Cook MC: Nurses' six rights for safe medication administration, *Mass Nurse* 69(6):8, 1999.

Ways to Prevent Medication Errors
Read all orders, instructions, and labels carefully.
Ask questions if you do not understand.
Do not allow anyone or anything to interrupt.
Double check all calculations.
Use at least two ways to identify the patient.
Identify and report system issues.
Learn as much as you can about the medication you administer.

DRUG INTERACTIONS
Drug–Drug Interactions
- Digoxin and thiazide diuretics (hypokalemia causes digoxin toxicity)
- Cimetidine and warfarin (warfarin is potentiated)
- Cimetidine and phenytoin (phenytoin blood level is increased)
- Quinolone antibiotics and warfarin (warfarin is potentiated)
- Nonsteroidal antiinflammatory drugs (NSAIDs) and diuretics (decreased effectiveness of diuretics)
- NSAIDs and aspirin (increased erosion of stomach lining)
- ACE inhibitors and potassium-sparing diuretics (hyperkalemia)
- Warfarin and aspirin or NSAIDs (increased action of warfarin)
- Fiber or bulk laxatives (inhibits absorption of any drug)
- Antacids (may inhibit absorption of medications)
- Phenytoin and magnesium-based antacids (decreased absorption of phenytoin)

Drug–Food Interactions
- Carbidopa or levodopa and protein (decreased absorption of drug)
- Cyclosporine and grapefruit juice (increased serum level of cyclosporine)
- Tetracycline and dairy products (decreased absorption of tetracycline)
- Quinolone antibiotics and dairy products (decreased absorption of drugs)
- Monoamine oxidase inhibitors and wine or cheese (causes severe hypertension)

- Sedatives and alcohol (increased sedation)
- Warfarin and psyllium (decreased absorption and decreased effectiveness of warfarin)
- Warfarin and vitamin E (increased effectiveness of warfarin)
- Iron tablets and tea, bran, or eggs (decreased absorption of iron)

Medications That May Contribute to Cognitive Impairment in Older Adults

Analgesics Codeine, meperidine, morphine, NSAIDs, propoxyphene

Antihistamines Diphenhydramine, hydroxyzine

Antihypertensives Clonidine, diuretics, hydralazine, methyldopa, propranolol

Anitmicrobials Gentamicin, isoniazid

Antiparkinson agents Amantadine, bromocriptine, carbidopa/levodopa

Cardiovascular drugs Atropine, digoxin, lidocaine, quinidine

Psychotropics Barbiturates, benzodiazepines, chlorpromazine, haloperidol, lithium, risperidone, selective serotonin reuptake inhibitor (SSRI) antidepressants, tricyclic antidepressants

Drug Actions in Older Adults		
Problem	Cause	Intervention
Difficulty swallowing medications	Loss of elasticity in oral mucosa	Rinse mouth before taking pills.
Erosion of esophageal tissues from pills	Delayed esophageal clearance	Position patient upright. Crush pill (if possible).
Stomach irritation from medications	Decreased gastric acidity or peristalsis	Drink a full glass of water. Take with food.
Slower drug absorption	Reduced colon muscle tone	Increase fluids. Avoid constipation.
Fragile veins	Reduced skin elasticity	Avoid IV punctures.
Slower drug metabolism	Reduced liver size	Monitor dosages.
	Reduced hepatic flow	Monitor liver effects.
Slower drug excretion	Reduced glomerular filtration	Monitor dosages. Monitor renal effects.

INFILTRATION AND PHLEBITIS SCALES
Infiltration Scale

Grade	Clinical Criteria
0	No symptoms
1	Skin blanched and cool to the touch
	Edema, <1 inch in any direction
	With or without pain
2	Skin blanched and cool to the touch
	Edema 1–6 inches in any direction
	With or without pain
3	Skin blanched, translucent, cool to touch
	Gross edema >6 inches in any direction
	Mild to moderate pain and possible numbness
4	Skin blanched, translucent, and tight; possible leaking
	Skin discolored, bruised, swollen
	Gross edema >6 inches in any direction
	Deep pitting tissue edema with circulatory impairment
	Moderate to severe pain
	Infiltration of any amount of blood product, irritant, or vesicant

Phlebitis Scale

Grade	Clinical Criteria
0	No symptoms
1	Erythema at access site with or without pain
2	Pain at access site with erythema, edema, or both
3	Pain at access site with erythema, edema, or both
	Streak formation with palpable venous cord
4	Pain access site with erythema, edema, or both
	Streak formation, Palpable venous cord >1 inch in length
	Purulent drainage

THERAPEUTIC DRUGS THAT REQUIRE SERUM DRUG LEVELS FOLLOWED BY AVERAGE RANGES*[†]

Antibiotics

Amikacin (Amikin) 15 to 25 mcg/mL
Gentamicin (Garamycin) 5 to 10 mcg/mL
Tobramycin (Nebcin) 5 to 10 mcg/mL

Anticonvulsants

Carbamazepine (Tegretol) 5 to 12 mcg/mL
Phenobarbital 10 to 30 mcg/mL

---

*Specific therapeutic blood levels may vary per facility.
[†]Other drugs may be included depending on the facility.

Phenytoin (Dilantin) 10 to 20 mcg/mL
Primidone (Mysoline) 5 to 12 mcg/mL
Valproic acid 50 to 100 mcg/mL

Antidepressants
Amitriptyline 120 to 150 ng/mL
Desipramine 150 to 300 ng/mL
Imipramine 150 to 300 ng/mL
Nortriptyline 50 to 150 ng/mL

Cardiovascular Drugs
Digoxin (Lanoxin) 0.8 to 2.0 ng/mL
Lidocaine (Xylocaine) 1.5 to 5.0 mcg/mL
Procainamide (Pronestyl) 4 to 10 mcg/mL
Propranolol 50 to 100 ng/mL
Quinidine and disopyramide 2 to 5 mcg/mL

Respiratory Drug
Theophylline (Aminophylline) 10 to 20 mcg/mL

DRUG ADMINISTRATION

Syringe Compatibility											
	Atropine	Buprenorphine	Butorphanol	Chlorpromazine	Codeine	Diazepam	Dimenhydrinate	Diphenhydramine	Droperidol	Fentanyl	Glycopyrrolate	Heparin
Atropine			C	C		I	C	C	C	C	C	
Buprenorphine												
Butorphanol	C			C		I	I	C	C	C		
Chlorpromazine	C		C			I	I	C	C	C	C	C
Codeine						I						
Diazepam	I		I	I	I		I	I	I	I	I	
Dimenhydrinate	C		I	I		I		C	C	C	I	
Diphenhydramine	C		C	C		I	C		C	C	C	
Droperidol	C		C	C		I	C	C		C	C	I
Fentanyl	C		C	C		I	C	C	C		C	
Glycopyrrolate	C			C		I	I	C	C	C		
Heparin			I	C		I			I			
Hydroxyzine	C		C	C		I	I	C	C	C	C	
Meperidine	C		C	C		I	C	C	C	C	C	I
Metoclopramide	C		C	C		I	C	C	C	C		
Midazolam	C		C	C			I	C	C	C	C	
Morphine	**C**		**C**	**C**		I	**C**	**C**	**C**	**C**	**C**	I
Nalbuphine*	C					I			C			
Pentazocine	C		C	C		I	C	C	C	C	I	I
Pentobarbital	C		I	I	I	I	I	I	I	I	I	
Perphenazine	C		C	C		I	C	C	C	C		
Prochlorperazine	C		C	C		I	I	C	C	C	C	
Promazine	C			C		I	I	C	C	C	C	
Promethazine	C		C	C		I	I	C	C	C	C	
Ranitidine	C			C			C	C		C	C	
Scopolamine Hbr	C		C	C		I	C	C	C	C	C	
Secobarbital	I		I	I	I	I	I	I	I	I	I	
Thiethylperazine			C			I						

*Compatibility depends on manufacturer, Wyeth and DuPont forms are incompatible.

Give within 15 minutes of mixing.

C = compatible; I = incompatible; □ = no documented information.

Syringe Compatibility—cont'd

Hydroxyzine	Meperidine	Metoclopramide	Midazolam	Morphine	Nalbuphine	Pentazocine	Pentobarbital	Perphenazine	Prochlorperazine	Promazine	Promethazine	Ranidine	Scopolamine Hbr	Secobarbital	Thiethylperazine
C	C	C	C	C	C	C	C	C	C	C	C	C	C	I	
C	C	C	C	C		C	I	C	C		C		C	I	C
C	C	C	C	C		C	I	C	C	C	C	C	C	I	
							I							I	
I	I	I		I	I	I	I	I	I	I	I		I	I	I
I	C	C	I	C		C	I	C	I	I	I	C	C	I	
C	C	C	C	C		C	I	C	C	C	C	C	C	I	
C	C	C		C	C	C	I	C	C	C	C		C	I	
C	C	C		C		C	I	C	C	C	C	C	C	I	
	I			I		I					I				
	C	C		C	C	C	I		C	C	C	I	C	I	
C		C		I		C	I	C	C	C	C	C	C	I	
C	C			C		C			C	C	C	C	C	I	
C		C		C	C		I	I	I	C	C	I	C		C
C	I	C				C	I	C	C	C	C	C	C	I	
C						I		C				C	C	I	C
C	C	C		C			I	C	C	C	C	C	C	I	
I	I			I	I	I		I	I	I	I		C	C	
	C	C		C		C	I		C		C	C	C	I	I
C	C	C		C	C	C	I	C		C	C	C	C	I	
C	C	C		C		C	I		C		C		C	I	
C	C	C		C	C	C	I	C	C	C		C	C	I	
	C	C	I	C	C	C		C	C		C		C		C
C	C	C		C	C	C	C	C	C	C	C	C		I	
I	I	I		I	I	I	I	I	I	I	I		I		I
					C				I				C		I

†Parenteral compatibility occurs when two or more drugs are successfully mixed without liquefaction, deliquescence, or precipitation.

From Skidmore-Roth L: *2012 Mosby's nursing drug reference*, ed 25, St. Louis, 2012, Mosby; Developed by Providence Memorial Hospital, El Paso, Texas.

Injection Guide for Needle Size and Volume

		Volume Injected (mL)	
	Needle Sizes	Average	Range
Intradermal	26 or 27 gauge × ⅜ in	0.1	0.0001–1.0
Subcutaneous	25–27 gauge × ½ to 1½ in	0.5	0.5–1.5
Intramuscular			
Gluteus medius	20–23 gauge × 1½ to 3 in	2–4	1–5
Gluteus minimus	20–23 gauge × 1½ to 3 in	1–4	1–5
Vastus lateralis	22–25 gauge × ⅝ to 1½ in	1–4	1–5
Deltoid	23–25 gauge × ⅝ to 1 in	0.5	0.5–2
Intravenous bolus	18–23 gauge× 1 to 1½ in	1–10	0.5–50 (or more by continuous infusion)

Flushing Venous Access Devices

Device	Solution/Volume	Frequency
Peripheral capped line	Normal saline (2–5 mL)	Daily 8 hours or after use and before use
Hickman or CVP	Heparinized or normal saline 10 units/mL (5 mL)	Daily or after each use
PICC or Cook catheter	Heparinized or normal saline 10 units/mL (5 mL)	Daily or after each use
Groshong catheter	Normal saline (10 mL) (20 mL with viscous Medication/blood)	Daily or after each use
Groshong implanted	Normal saline (10 mL)	Daily or after each use
Per-Q-Catheter	Heparinized or normal saline 10 units/mL (5 mL)	Every or after each use

Continued

| | Flushing Venous Access Devices—cont'd | |
Device	Solution/Volume	Frequency
Gesco catheter	Heparinized or normal saline 10 units/mL (5 mL)	Daily or after each use
Midline-L/Luther Cath (should not use for blood draws)	Heparinized or normal saline 10 units/mL (5 mL)	Daily or after each use
Implanted port (chest)	Huber-type needle Heparinized or normal saline 100 units/mL (5 mL)	Every month or after each use
PAS port (arm)	Heparinized or normal saline 10 units/mL (5 mL) Normal saline (20 mL)	Daily or after each use After blood draws

CVP, Central venous pressure; PAS, peripherally accessed system; PICC, peripherally inserted central catheter.
Flushing policies may vary per facility and may require a physician order

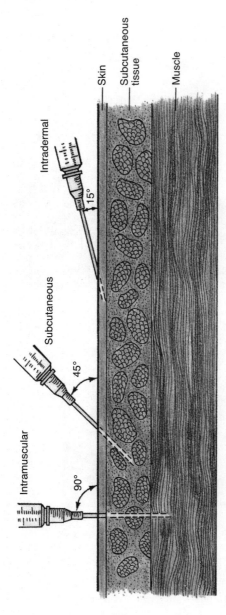

Figure 2-1 Comparison of the angles of insertion of intramuscular, subcutaneous, and intradermal injections. (From Potter PA, Perry AG, Stockert PA, Hall A: *Fundamentals of nursing,* ed 8, St. Louis, 2013, Mosby.)

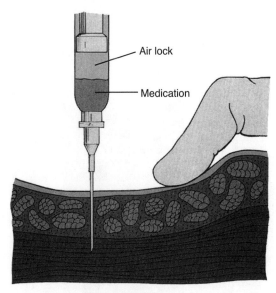

During injection

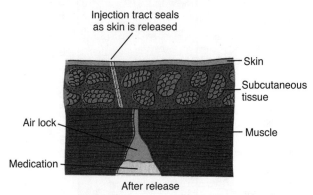

After release

Figure 2-2 A, Pull on overlying skin during
intramuscular injection moves tissues to prevent later
tracking. **B,** Z track left after injection prevents deposit
of medication through sensitive tissue. (From Potter PA,
Perry AG: *Fundamentals of nursing,* ed 7, St. Louis, 2009,
Mosby.)

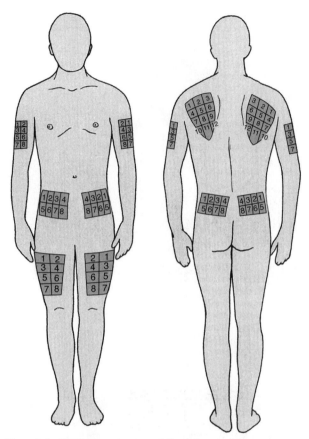

Figure 2-3 Common sites used for subcutaneous injections. (From Potter PA, Perry AG, Stockert PA, Hall A: *Fundamentals of nursing,* ed 8, St. Louis, 2013, Mosby.)

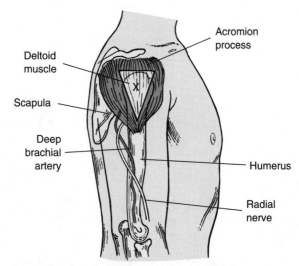

Figure 2-4 Deltoid injections. (From Potter PA, Perry AG, Stockert PA, Hall A: *Fundamentals of nursing*, ed 8, St. Louis, 2013, Mosby.)

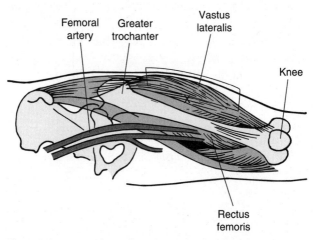

Figure 2-5 Vastus lateralis injections. (From Potter PA, Perry AG, Stockert PA, Hall A: *Fundamentals of nursing*, ed 8, St. Louis, 2013, Mosby.)

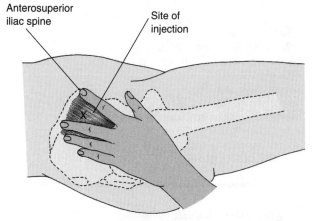

Figure 2-6 Ventrogluteal injections. (From Potter PA, Perry AG, Stockert PA, Hall A: *Fundamentals of nursing,* ed 8, St. Louis, 2013, Mosby.)

CHAPTER 3

Infection Control

For an in-depth study of infection control, consult the following publications:

Hospital Infection Control Practices Advisory Committee, Centers for Disease Control and Prevention: *Guidelines for isolation precautions in hospitals*, Washington, DC, 1996, Public Health Service, US Department of Health and Human Services.

Potter PA, Perry AG, Stockert PA, Hall A: *Fundamentals of nursing*, ed 8, St. Louis, 2013, Mosby.

Universal precautions for prevention of transmission of human immunodeficiency virus, hepatitis B virus, and other bloodborne pathogens in health care settings, *MMWR Morbid Mortal Wkly Rep* 37(suppl 24):377, 1988.

BASIC TERMINOLOGY

Asepsis Prevention of the transfer of microorganisms and pathogens

Chain Path of infection; the components of the infectious disease process

Clean Presence of few microorganisms or pathogens with no visible debris

Colonization Presence of a potentially infectious organism in or on a host but not causing disease

Communicable Ability of a microorganism to spread disease

Contamination Presence of an infectious agent on a surface

Dirty Presence of many microorganisms or pathogens; any soiled item

Disease Alteration of normal tissues, body processes, or functions

Etiology Cause of a disease

Immunity Resistance to a disease associated with the presence of antibodies

Infection Invasion of tissues by a disease-causing microorganism(s)

Medical asepsis Measures that limit pathologic spread of microorganisms

Nosocomial infection A hospital-acquired infection (not present or incubating on admission)

Ports How microorganisms exit and enter a system

Reservoir Storage place for organisms to grow

Source Point that initiates chain of infection

Sterile Absence of all microorganisms

Surgical asepsis Measures to keep pathogenic organisms at a minimum during surgery

Transmission Method by which microorganisms travel from one host to another

Virulence Ability of a microorganism to produce disease

STAGES OF INFECTION

Incubation From initial contact with infectious material to onset of symptoms

Prodrome From nonspecific signs and symptoms to specific signs and symptoms (prodromal)

Illness Presence of specific signs and symptoms

Convalescence During the recovery period as symptoms subside

THE INFLAMMATORY PROCESS

Stage I

Constriction of blood vessels, dilatation of small vessels, increased vessel permeability, increased leukocytes, swelling, and pain. Leukocytes begin to engulf the infection.

Stage II

Exudation with fluids and dead cells

Serous Clear; part of the blood

Purulent Thick; pus with leukocytes

Sanguineous Bloody

Stage III

Repair of tissues. Examples include:

Regeneration Same tissues

Stroma Connective tissues

Parenchyma Functional part

Fibrous Scar

SUMMARY OF ISOLATION PRECAUTIONS

Handwashing Should be done before and after working with all patients and after removing gloves; immediately if hands become contaminated with blood or other body fluids

Gloves Should be worn whenever contact with body fluids is likely

Mask and/or eye cover Should be worn when splashing of body fluids is likely

Gown Should be worn when soiling of exposed skin or clothing is likely

CPR Should be done with pocket masks or mechanical ventilation, avoiding mouth to mouth

Needles Should not be recapped unless using the one-handed method and *only* if procedure indicates recapping is needed; needles should have safety guards

CAUTION: *Do not break needles; discard all sharp objects immediately.*

Private rooms Should be used whenever possible

Spills Should be cleaned immediately with bleach and water (one part bleach to nine parts water) for FDA-approved cleaning agent

Specimens Should be collected in leakproof, puncture-resistant container; outside of container must be free of contaminants

Transporting patients Should be kept to a minimum when working with infected patients

TYPES OF ISOLATION PRECAUTIONS
Standard Precautions
- Used to help prevent nosocomial infections
- Used when working with all patients
- Replaces the universal precautions and the blood and body precautions
- Applies to blood, all body fluids, secretions, excretions (except sweat)
- To be used even if blood is not visible
- Also applies to nonintact skin and mucous membranes
- Designed to reduce the risk of transmission of microorganisms

Transmission-Based Precautions
- Used for patients known or suspected to be infected with specific pathogens
- There are three subgroups of transmission-based precautions.
- Subgroups can be combined for diseases with multiple transmissions routes.
- Subgroups are to be used in addition to standard precautions.

Airborne Precautions
Used for airborne infectious agents of 5 micrometers or smaller

Droplet Precautions
- Used for infectious agents larger than 5 micrometers
- Droplets from the mucous membranes of the nose or mouth
- Droplets from coughing, sneezing, or talking
- Droplet contracted within 3 feet or less

Contact Precautions
Contact can be direct or indirect:
- Direct is skin-to-skin contact through touch, turning, or bathing.
- Indirect contact is made by touching contaminated items, items within the patient's room.

CDC GUIDELINES FOR HAND HYGIENE IN HEALTH CARE SETTINGS (2002)
Indications for handwashing and hand antisepsis
- When hands are visibly dirty or contaminated
- Before and after having direct contact with patients

- Before donning sterile gloves when inserting a central intravascular catheter
- Before inserting indwelling urinary catheters, peripheral vascular catheters, or other invasive devices that do not require a surgical procedure
- After contact with a patient's intact skin
- After contact with body fluids or excretions, mucous membranes, nonintact skin, and wound dressings if hands are not visibly soiled
- If moving from a contaminated body site to a clean body site during patient care
- After contact with inanimate objects (including medical equipment) in the immediate vicinity of the patient
- After removing gloves
- Before eating and after using a restroom

ANTIBIOTIC-RESISTANT PATHOGENS

Acinetobacter baumannii Multidrug-resistance (MRAB)

Clostridium difficile Clindamycin resistant; fluoroquinolone-resistant Cipro (ciprofloxacin) and Levaquin (levofloxacin)

Escherichia coli 80% of the bacteria are resistant to one or more drugs

Enterococcus Vancomycin-resistant (VRE see p. 69)

Mycobacterium tuberculosis Multiple-drug resistant (MDR-TB)

Salmonella Resistant to nine different antibiotics

Staphylococcus aureus Methicillin resistant (MRSA see p. 68), linezolid resistant, vancomycin resistant (VRSA); CA-MRSA (community-acquired MRSA)

Streptococcus pyogenes (group A strep) Macrolide resistant

Streptococcus pneumoniae Penicillin resistant

PREVENTION OF RESISTANT PATHOGENS

*   Wash hand and use alcohol-based hand sanitizes to reduce the spread of bacteria.
*   Adhere to all organizational infection control policy and procedures.
*   Use patient-specific equipment for patients when possible.
*   Clean environmental surfaces regularly and when soiled.
*   Use personal protective equipment (PPE) according to facility's infection control policy.
*   Use antibiotics only when needed and complete each course of antibiotics as prescribed.

MRSA AND VRE

MRSA Methicillin-resistant *Staphylococcus aureus*

VRE Vancomycin-resistant *Enterococcus*

These are two of the most difficult infections to treat.

USE **CONTACT PRECAUTIONS** for a skin or body fluid, MRSA, or VRE infection.

USE **DROPLET PRECAUTIONS** for a respiratory MRSA infection and for when MRSA is found in tracheal secretions.

Always wash hands with chlorhexidine gluconate soap before entering and after leaving each patient's room.

Standard Precautions for MRSA

Masks Necessary if patient's respiratory tract is colonized or has an active infection; must use when suctioning or when patient has a productive cough

Gowns Necessary if in contact with secretions

Gloves Necessary for all contact with items that may be contaminated

Private room If possible or with other patients with MRSA and no other infections

Standard Precautions for VRE

Masks Necessary if contact with secretions is likely

Gowns Necessary if contact with secretions is likely

Gloves Necessary for all contact with items that may be contaminated

Private room If possible or with patients who have VRE and no other infections

COMMON BACTERIA

These are normal flora found on or in the body.

Ear *Corynebacterium*, diphtheroids, saprophytes, *Staphylococcus, Streptococcus*

Esophagus and stomach None; usually microorganisms from the mouth or food

Eye Corynebacterium, *Enterobacter, Haemophilus, Moraxella, Neisseria, Staphylococcus, Streptococcus*

Genitalia *Bacteroides, Candida albicans, Corynebacterium, Enterococcus, Fusobacterium, Mycobacterium, Mycoplasma, Neisseria, Staphylococcus, Streptococcus*

Ileum (lower) *Bacteroides, Clostridium, Enterobacter, Enterococcus, Lactobacillus, Mycobacterium, Staphylococcus*

Ileum (upper) *Enterococcus, Lactobacillus*
Large intestine *Acinetobacter, Actinomyces, Alcaligenes, Bacteroides, Clostridium, Enterobacter, Enterococcus, Eubacterium, Fusobacterium, Mycobacterium, Peptococcus, Peptostreptococcus*
Mouth *Actinomyces, Bacteroides, Candida albicans, Corynebacterium, Enterobacter,* Fusobacterium, *Lactobacillus, Peptococcus, Peptostreptococcus, Staphylococcus, Streptococcus, Torulopsis, Veillonella*
Nose *Corynebacterium, Enterobacter, Haemophilus, Moraxella, Neisseria, Staphylococcus, Streptococcus*
Oropharynx *Corynebacterium, Enterobacter, Haemophilus, Staphylococcus, Streptococcus*
Skin Bacillus, *Candida albicans, Corynebacterium,* dermatophytes, *Enterobacter, Peptococcus, Propionibacterium acnes, Staphylococcus, Streptococcus*

TUBERCULOSIS
Agent
- *Mycobacterium tuberculosis* (Note that some strains are becoming resistant to antibiotics.)
- Bovine TB (*Mycobacterium bovis*), which is transmitted through cattle and unpasteurized milk

Reservoir
- Primarily humans
- Diseased cattle
- Badgers
- Other small mammals

Mode of Transmission
- Spread by respiratory droplets
- Direct invasion through mucous membranes

Incubation
- 4 to 12 weeks
- Subsequent risk of pulmonary infection is greatest within the first year
- Injections may persist for a lifetime

Prevention
- Education regarding the mode of transmission and early diagnosis
- Monitoring of groups at risk (people who are HIV positive, recent immigrants, homeless people, people residing in crowded substandard housing)
- Report new cases for public health follow-up
- Implement standard precautions and transmission-based airborne precautions immediately with any suspected cases (see p. 65)
- Eliminate tuberculosis among dairy cattle
- Pasteurize milk

OVERVIEW OF COMMON INFECTIOUS DISEASES
- Standard precautions are required for all persons with infectious diseases (see p. 65).
- Check state requirements for reporting infectious diseases.

AIDS
Transmission through blood and body fluids, sexual contact, sharing IV needles, contaminated blood, and from mother to fetus

Considerations Education regarding mode of transmission, avoidance of sexual contact with infected persons, use of latex condoms, proper blood screening of all transfusable products, and proper handling of needles and other contaminated material

Chickenpox/Herpes Zoster Virus (Varicella/Shingles)
Transmission through respiratory droplets or by direct contact with open lesions
Considerations Contact isolation, avoid direct contact with lesions, and administration of varicella zoster immune globulin. Caregivers should be chickenpox immune. **New vaccines are available.**

Chlamydia
Transmission through sexual contact
Considerations Public education; use of latex condoms

German Measles (Rubella)
Transmission through respiratory droplets
Considerations Education regarding vaccines and prenatal care; avoidance of contact

Gonorrhea
Transmission through vaginal secretions, semen, sexual contact
Considerations Public education regarding mode of transmission; use of latex condoms. Some strains are antibiotic resistant.

Hepatitis A and Hepatitis E
Transmission through direct contact with water, food, or feces
Considerations Handwashing before touching food, proper water and sewage treatment, reporting of cases, immunoglobulin vaccination when traveling to high-risk areas, proper disposal of contaminants

Hepatitis B
Transmission through all fluids of an infected source

Considerations Hepatitis B vaccination, public education, blood screening, use of gloves when handling secretions, proper sterilization of equipment, reporting of all known cases

Hepatitis C
Transmission through contaminated blood, plasma, and needles

Considerations See Hepatitis B.

Hepatitis D
Hepatitis D can develop only in individuals who have active hepatitis B and in those who are carriers of hepatitis D.

Measles (Red, Hard, Morbilli, Rubeola)
Transmission through airborne droplets or direct contact with lesions

Considerations Public education about vaccine; avoidance of contact with infected persons

Meningitis (Bacterial)
Transmission through airborne droplets or direct contact

Considerations Public education, vaccination; early prophylaxis of exposed contacts

Mononucleosis
Transmission through saliva

Considerations Public education; good hygiene

Mumps
Transmission through airborne droplets and saliva

Consideration Vaccination

Pneumonia
Transmission through airborne droplets
Considerations Vaccination; good hygiene; some
    strains are antibiotic resistant

Polio (Poliomyelitis)
Transmission through oral or fecal contact
Consideration Vaccination

Salmonellosis
Transmission through ingestion of contaminated
food
Considerations Proper cooking and storage
    of food; good handwashing before food
    preparation

Syphilis
Transmission through sexual contact, direct contact
with lesions, and blood transfusions
Considerations Public education regarding
    transmission, prenatal screening, and prenatal
    follow-up; use of latex condoms; blood
    screening

Tetanus (Lockjaw)
Transmission through direct contact of wounds
with infected soil or feces
Considerations Public education regarding mode
    of transmission, vaccination

Tuberculosis
Transmission through airborne droplets; bovine TB
through unpasteurized milk
Considerations Public education and screening,
    improvement of overcrowded living conditions,
    and pasteurization of milk

Typhoid Fever
Transmission through contaminated water, urine, or feces
Considerations Good hygiene, sanitary water, proper sewage care, and vaccinations

Whooping Cough (Pertussis)
Transmission through airborne droplets and nasal discharge
Considerations Vaccination, wearing of masks when near infected patients, reporting of all cases

FACTS ABOUT INFLUENZA
- Symptoms include fever, headache, dry mouth, fatigue, sore throat, and muscle aches.
- Up to 20% of Americans get the flu each year.
- Influenza in conjunction with pneumonia is the sixth leading cause of death in the United States among older adults.
- A person cannot catch influenza from a vaccine.
- Because influenza viruses can change from year to year, an annual influenza shot is needed each fall.
- The best time to receive an influenza vaccine is October through December.
- Influenza vaccine will not protect from other illnesses, such as colds, bronchitis, and the stomach influenza or gastritis.
- Vaccinations can prevent up to 50% of the 140,000 hospitalizations and 80% of the 300,000 deaths that occur each year.
- Influenza can worsen heart and lung diseases and diabetes.
- Influenza can lead to pneumonia.

Facts about Pneumococcal Disease in Adults

- An infection or inflammation of the lungs.
- In conjunction with influenza, it is the seventh leading cause of death in the United States.
- Several different causes, including bacterial, viral, fungal, mycoplasmas, and chemical.
- *Streptococcus pneumoniae* is the most common cause of bacterial pneumonia. It is one form of pneumonia for which a vaccine is available.
- Half of all pneumonias are believed to be caused by viruses.
- Viral pneumonias may be complicated by an invasion of bacteria with all the typical symptoms of bacterial pneumonia.
- The greatest risk of pneumococcal pneumonia is usually among people who have chronic illnesses of the lung or heart, sickle cell anemia, diabetes, recovering from illness, or those older than age 65 years.
- Prevented by the use of vaccines usually given at age 65 or younger for persons who smoke or have an underlying medical condition.
- A person cannot catch pneumococcal diseases from a vaccine.
- Vaccine can be given any time of the year.
- Vaccine can be given at the same time is the influenza vaccine.
- Pneumococcal and Shingles vaccines should not be given during the same medical visit.

Courtesy of National Foundation for Infectious Diseases.

Specimen Collection Techniques

Amount Needed*	Collection Device	Specimen Collection and Transport
	Wound Culture	
Only with normal saline	Sterile cotton-tipped swab or syringe	Place sterile test tube or culturette tube on clean paper towel. After swabbing center of wound site, grasp collection tube by holding it with paper towel. Carefully insert swab without touching outside of tube. After washing hands and securing tube's top, transfer labeled tube into bag for transport to laboratory.

Continued

	Specimen Collection Techniques—cont'd	
Amount Needed*	**Collection Device**	**Specimen Collection and Transport**
	Blood Culture	
10 mL per culture bottle from two different venipuncture sites (volume may differ based on collection containers)	Syringes and culture media bottles	Perform venipuncture at two different sites to decrease likelihood of both specimens being contaminated by skin flora. Wash hands. Cleanse area per facility policy. Inject 10 mL of blood into each bottle. Secure tops of bottles, label specimens per facility policy, and send to laboratory.
	Stool Culture	
Small amount, approximately the size of a walnut	Clean cup with seal top (not necessary to be sterile) and tongue blade	Using tongue blade, collect needed amount of feces from bedpan. Transfer feces to cup without touching cup's outside surface. Wash hands and place seal on cup. Label specimen. Transfer specimen cup into clean bag for transport to laboratory.

Urine Culture

1–5 mL	Syringe and sterile cup	Use syringe to collect specimen if patient has Foley catheter. Have patient follow procedure to obtain clean-voided specimen if not catheterized. Transfer urine into sterile container by injecting urine from syringe or pouring it from used container. Wash hands and secure top of labeled container. Transfer labeled specimen into clean bag for transport to laboratory.

*Agency policies may differ on type of containers, amount of specimen material required, and bagging. From Potter PA, Perry AG, Stockert PA, Hall A: *Fundamentals of nursing*, ed 8, St. Louis, 2013, Mosby.

TYPES OF IMMUNITY

Active Antibodies produced in body; long lasting
- **Natural** Antibodies produced during an active infection
  - *Examples:* Chickenpox, mumps, measles
- **Artificial** Vaccine of actual antigens
  - *Examples:* Mumps measles, rubella (MMR)

Passive Antibodies produced outside the body; short acting
- **Natural** Antibodies passed from mother to child through placenta and breast milk
- **Artificial** Injected immune serum

ANTIBODY FUNCTIONS

IgM First to respond; activates the complement system; stimulates ingestion by macrophage; principal antibody of the blood

IgG Most prevalent antibody; major antibody of the tissues; produced after IgM; only antibody to cross placenta; antitoxin; antiviral

IgA Principal antibody of the GI tract; found in tears, saliva, sweat, breast milk; protects epithelial lining

IgD Only in minute concentrations; function unknown

IgE For allergic reactions

CHAPTER 4

Basic Nursing Assessments

For an in-depth study of basic nursing assessments, consult the following publications:

Lewis SM, et al: *Medical-surgical nursing*, ed 8, St. Louis, 2011, Mosby.
Nugent P, Green J, Hellmer Saul MA, Pelikan P: *Mosby's comprehensive review of nursing for the NCLEX-RN examination*, ed 20, St. Louis, 2012, Mosby.
Potter PA, Perry AG, Stockert PA, Hall A: *Fundamentals of nursing*, ed 8, St. Louis, 2013, Mosby.
Weilitz P, Potter PA: *Pocket guide for health assessment*, ed 6, St. Louis, 2007, Mosby.

THE PATIENT INTERVIEW
Demographics
Includes name, address, sex, age, birth date, marital status or significant other, religion, race, education, occupation, hobbies, significant life events

Health History
Includes history of smoking, heart disease, alcohol or other drug use or abuse, surgeries, injuries, childhood diseases and vaccinations, hypertension, diabetes, arthritis, seizures, cancer, emotional problems, transfusions, drug or food allergies, perception of patient's health or illness, lifestyle, hygiene and eating habits, health practices

Family Medical History
Includes history of heart disease, alcohol or drug use or abuse, diabetes, arthritis, cancer, emotional problems

Current Situation
Reasons for seeking help or chief complaint; include annual check-up, follow-up care, second opinion, new symptoms, monitoring existing health problem(s)

History of Present Illness
Includes location and quality of symptoms, chronology, aggravating and alleviating factors, associated symptoms, effect on lifestyle, measures used to deal with symptoms, review of body systems

Medications
Prescribed, occasional use (CPRN), over the counter, herbals

FUNCTIONAL ASSESSMENT
Health Perceptions
General health (good, fair, poor)
Tobacco or alcohol use (how much, how long)
Recreational or prescribed medications (list)
Hygiene practices

Nutrition
Type of diet (list)
Enjoys snacks (yes/no, what type)
Fluid intake (types of fluids)
Fluid restriction (yes/no)
Skin (normal, dry, rash)
Teeth (own, dentures, bridge)
Weight (recent gain or loss)

Respiration and Circulation
Respiratory problems (shortness of breath)
Smoking history
Circulation problems (chest pain, edema,
    pacemaker)

Elimination
Upper GI (nausea, vomiting, dysphagia,
    discomfort)
Bowels (frequency, consistency, last bowel
    movement, ostomy)
Bladder (incontinence, dysuria, urgency, frequency,
    nocturia, hematuria)

Activity and Exercise
Energy level (high, normal, low)
Usual exercise and activity patterns (recent
    changes)
Needs assistance with (eating, bathing, dressing)
Requirements (cane, walker, wheelchair, crutches)

Sleep
Problems (falling asleep, early waking, hours per
   night, napping)
Methods used to facilitate sleep
Feelings on waking (fatigued, refreshed)

Cognitive
Educational level
Learning needs
Communication barriers (list)
Memory loss (yes/no)
Developmental age
Reads English (yes/no)
Other languages (list)

Sensory
Hearing and vision (no problems, impaired,
   devices)
Pain (yes/no, how managed)

Coping and Stress
Needs (social services, financial counselor)
May need (home care, nursing home)
Coping mechanisms used by patient

Self-Perception
How illness or wellness is affecting patient
Body image or self-esteem concerns

Roles and Relationships
Significant other or emergency contacts
Primary, secondary, or tertiary roles
Role changes caused by illness or wellness
Role conflicts caused by illness or wellness

Sexuality
Last menstrual period, menopause, breast
   examination

Testicular examination
How illness may affect sexuality
How hospitalization may affect sexuality
Any questions, needs, or additional concerns

Values and Beliefs
Religious or cultural affiliation
Religious or cultural beliefs concerning health or
    illness
Holiday or food restrictions while hospitalized
Religious or cultural restrictions on medications or
    treatments
Religious or cultural rituals needed while
    hospitalized
Clergy or religious leader requested while
    hospitalized

INTERVIEWING STRATEGIES
Open-ended questions: "How can I help you?"
Summarizing statements: "Coughing and wheezing
    seem to be your concerns."
Reflective statements: "You seem out of breath."
Leading questions: "Is your sputum green?"
Focused questions: "Are you short of breath
    now?"
Clarification: "When did you last take you
    inhaler?"
Restating: "So you said your shortness of breath
    became worse yesterday?"
Encouraging: "Tell me more about your
    breathing."

CULTURAL ASSESSMENT
Include introductory information, such as:
• Patient's name, unit, or room number
• Admission date, admitting diagnosis
• Proposed length of stay

Information about the country can be important:

- What is the cultural or ethnic affiliation?
- In what country was the patient born?
- How many years has he or she been in the United States?
- What generation American is the patient?

Assess language needs:

- Does the patient need an interpreter (what language)?
- Does the patient need a communication tool (language board)?
- Could the patient use telephone language line (available through most local telephone companies)?

Assess for cultural practices:

- Are there special rituals that may need to be honored?
- Are there special health practices that may need to be honored?
- How will the illness affect cultural practices?
- How will the illness affect cultural rituals?

Assess for cultural supports:

- Which cultural or ethnic supports may help your patient?
- To whom does the patient turn for help?
- How does the patient describe his or her family?
- Who is the patient's main source of support?
- Who is the patient's main source of hope?

SPIRITUAL ASSESSMENT

Include introductory information, such as:

- Patient's name, unit, or room number
- Admission date, admitting diagnosis
- Proposed length of stay
- Religious affiliation
- Local clergy and telephone number

Assess for potential religious supports:
- Minister, priest, rabbi, shaman, emmen, other
- The need for church or prayer services
- The need for confession, communion, religious music
- The need for a Bible, Koran, Bhagavad-Gita, prayer books

Assess for religious practices:
- Are there special rituals that may need to be honored?
- Are there special health practices that may need to be honored?
- Are there special religious dietary needs?
- Is there a special prayer schedule that should be followed?
- Are there special fasting rituals that should be followed?
- How will the illness affect religious practices?
- How will the illness affect religious rituals?

Assess for religious supports:
- Which religious supports may help your patient?
- To whom does the patient turn for help?
- How does the patient describe his or her family?
- Who is the patient's main source of support?
- Who is the patient's main source of hope?
- Where does your patient turn for comfort?
- What gives your patient's life meaning?
- Does your patient believe that the illness is a punishment?

PHYSICAL ASSESSMENT
Appearance
Stage of development, general health, striking features, height, weight, behavior, posture, communication skills, grooming, hygiene

Skin
Color, consistency, temperature, turgor, integrity, texture, lesions, mucous membranes

Hair
Color, texture, amount, distribution

Nails
Color, texture, shape, size

Neurologic
Pupil reaction, motor and verbal responses, gait, reflexes, neurologic checks

Musculoskeletal
Range of motion, gait, tone, posture

Cardiovascular
Heart rate and rhythm, Homans' sign, peripheral pulses and temperature, edema

Respiratory
Rate, rhythm, depth, effort, quality, expansion, cough, breath sounds, sputum (production, color, and amount), tracheostomy size, nasal patency

Gastrointestinal
Abdominal contour, bowel sounds, nausea, vomiting, ostomy type and care, fecal frequency, consistency, presence of blood

Genitourinary
Urine color; character, amount, odor, ostomy

Classification of Percussion Sounds			
Sound	**Pitch**	**Duration**	**Example**
Flat	High	Short	Muscle
Dull	Medium	Medium	Liver, heart
Resonant	Low	Long	Lungs
Hyperresonant	Lower	Longer	Emphysemic lungs
Tympanic	Lowest	Longest	Stomach, colon

ASSESSMENT TECHNIQUES

Inspection By visual or auditory observation
Auscultation By listening to sounds with a stethoscope
Palpation By touching
    Fingertips: Best for texture, moisture, shape
    Palmar surface of fingers: Best for vibration
    Dorsum of hand: Best for temperature
Percussion By striking the body and assessing the sound
    Light percussion: Best for tenderness, density
    Sharp percussion: Best for reflexes

TEMPERATURE

Normal Oral Averages		
	°C	**°F**
Infant	36–38	97–100
Child	37	98.6
Adult	37	98.6
Elderly adult	36	98

Time Required for Reading Glass Thermometer
Oral: 3 to 5 minutes
Axillary: 9 to 10 minutes
Rectal: 2 to 4 minutes

Time Required for Reading Disposable Thermometer
Hold the thermometer in place until the chemically impregnated dots change color (≈45 seconds).

Time Required for Reading Electronic Thermometer
Hold the thermometer in place until the light or auditory signal indicates a reading.

Time Required for Reading Tympanic Thermometer
Hold the thermometer in place until the reading is displayed (≈2 seconds).

Distance of Insertion for Rectal Thermometer
Child: 1 inch
Adult: $1\frac{1}{2}$ inches

Conversion Used for Fahrenheit
Axillary: Oral minus 1°F
Rectal: Oral plus 1°F

Factors Affecting Temperature
Age Infants and elderly adults respond drastically to change in temperature.
Exercise Increase exercise will increase heat production.
Hormones Fluctuations in hormones can cause fluctuations in temperature.
Stress Physical and emotional stress can increase body temperature.

Advantages and Disadvantages of Temperature Measurement Methods

Axilla

Advantages	Disadvantages
Safe, inexpensive, and noninvasive	Takes a long time
Can be used with newborns and unconscious patients	Not good for rapid changes

Disposable

Advantages	Disadvantages
Safe	May be less accurate
Noninvasive	More expensive
Comfortable	
Helpful for those in isolations	

Electronic

Advantages	Disadvantages
Rapid measurement, usually 4 seconds	May be less accurate
Ideal for children, unbreakable	Risk of transferring nosocomial infections

Mercury

Advantages	Disadvantages
Accessible to patients at home	Risk of breakage
Inexpensive and easy to store	Risk of mercury exposure

Continued

Advantages and Disadvantages of Temperature Measurement Methods—cont'd

Oral

Advantages	Disadvantages
Comfortable, accurate, easy to obtain Reflects rapid change in core temperature	Not recommended for those who have had oral surgery or who have epilepsy

Rectal

Advantages	Disadvantages
Very reliable	May lag behind core temperature during rapid changes Should not be used for those with diarrhea or who have had rectal surgery

Skin

Advantages	Disadvantages
Safe, inexpensive, and noninvasive Can be used on neonates	Lags behind other sites during rapid temperature changes

Tympanic

Advantages	Disadvantages
Safe, inexpensive, and noninvasive Accurate and rapid measurement	Cannot be used with hearing aides Otitis media can distort readings

Special Factors

Circadian rhythm Lower temperatures in
morning; higher in afternoon

Hormones Progesterone will raise temperature.

Emotions Anxiety will raise temperature.

Clinical Signs of Fever

Onset Increased heart rate, increased respirations,
pallor, cool skin, cyanosis, chills, decreased
sweating, increased temperature

Course Flushed, warm skin; increased heart rate
and respiration; increased thirst; mild
dehydration; drowsiness; restlessness; decreased
appetite; weakness

Abatement Flushed skin, decreased shivering,
dehydration, diaphoresis

Fever Patterns

Fungal (infection) Rises slowly and stays high

Intermittent Spikes but falls to normal each day

Persistent or sustained Either remains elevated
or low grade; often caused by tumors of the
central nervous system

Relapsing Febrile for several days, alternating with
normal temperatures; often caused by parasites
or urinary tract infections

Remittent Spikes and falls but not to normal;
often noted with abscesses, tuberculosis, or
influenza viruses

Septic (infection) Wide peak and nadir, often
rigors and diaphoresis; often caused by gram-
negative organisms

THERMAL DISORDERS

Normal body temperature 37°C or 98.6°F

Frostbite Damage is caused to skin caused by
extreme cold. At or below 0°C (32°F), blood
vessels close to the skin constrict.
Treatment: Warm slowly.

Heatstroke Temperature above 42.2°C or 108°F
Treatment: Ice to groin and axilla.
Heat cramps Spasms of muscles
Treatment: Replace fluids; watch for chilling.
Hyperthermia Any temperature above
normal; severe hyperthermia is indicated
by temperatures at or above 42.2°C or
108°F.
Treatment: Replace fluids, watch for chilling.

Hypothermia (Stages)

Stage 1 Body temperature drops by 1°C to 2°C
(1.8°–3.6°F). Shivering occurs. Unable to
perform complex tasks with the hands. Blood
vessels in the outer extremities contract.
Breathing becomes quick and shallow. Goose
bumps form to create an insulating layer of air
around the body.
Stage 2 Body temperature drops by 2°C to 4°C
(3.6°F–7.2°F). Shivering becomes violent. Muscle
miscoordination becomes apparent. Mild
confusion, although the victim may appear alert.
Victim becomes pale. Lips, ears, fingers, and toes
may become blue.
Stage 3 Body temperature drops below
approximately 32°C or 90°F. Shivering may stop,
difficulty speaking, sluggish thinking, and
amnesia appear; inability to use hands and
stumbling are usually present. Skin becomes
blue and puffy, muscle coordination very poor,
walking nearly impossible, and the victim
exhibits incoherent or irrational behavior. Pulse
and respiration rates decrease, but Variable heart
rates (ventricular tachycardia, atrial fibrillation)
can occur. Major organs fail.
Treatment: Warm slowly.

WHEN TO MEASURE VITAL SIGNS
- On admission and discharge
- Before and after all procedures and diagnostic tests
- Before, during, and after medications that affect cardiovascular or respiratory functions
- When the patients reports onset or change in symptoms or any physical distress.

Temperature Conversions*		
°F–°C	°F–°C	°F–°C
95.0–35.0	100.2–37.9	105.1–40.6
95.2–35.1	**100.4–38.0**	105.4–40.8
95.4–35.2	100.6–38.1	105.6–40.9
95.5–35.3	100.8–38.2	**105.8–41.0**
95.7–35.4	101.0–38.3	106.0 41.1
95.9–35.5	101.1–38.4	106.2–41.2
96.1–35.6	101.3–38.5	106.3–41.3
96.3–35.7	101.5–38.6	106.5–41.4
96.6–35.9	101.7–38.7	106.7–41.5
96.8–36.0	102.0–38.8	106.9–41.6
97.0–36.1	**102.2–39.0**	107.2–41.8
97.2–36.2	102.4–39.1	107.4–41.9
97.3–36.3	102.6–39.2	**107.6–42.0**
97.5–36.4	102.8–39.3	107.8–42.1
97.7–36.5	103.0–39.4	108.0–42.2
97.9–36.5	103.1–39.5	108.1–42.3
98.2–36.8	103.3–39.6	108.3–42.4
98.4–36.9	103.6–39.8	108.5–42.5
98.6–37.0	103.8–39.9	108.7–42.6
98.8–37.1	**104.0–40.0**	109.0–42.7
98.9–37.2	104.2–40.1	109.2–42.9

Continued

Temperature Conversions—cont'd		
°F–°C	°F–°C	°F–°C
99.1–37.3	104.4–40.2	109.4–43.0
99.4–37.3	104.5–40.3	109.6–43.1
99.5–37.5	104.7–40.4	109.8–43.2
100.0–37.8	**105.0–40.5**	109.9–43.3

*To convert to Fahrenheit: $F = (C \times 9/5) + 32$.
To convert to Celsius: $C = (F - 32) \times 5/9$.
Key Temperatures are bolded

PULSE

Normal Ranges with Averages
Infant: 90–(140)–160 beats per minute
Child: 80–(100)–120 beats per minute
Adult: Women: 60–(80)–100 beats per minute;
      Men: 55–(75)–95 beats per minute

Assessments
Volume and Amplitude of Peripheral Pulses
 0 = Absent
1+ = Diminished/Barely palpable
2+ = Normal/Expected
3+ = Full/Strong
4+ = Bounding

Rhythm
Regular Normal
Regular or irregular Usually regular but
  occasionally irregular
Bigeminal Skips every other beat (monitor needed
  for detection)
Pulsus paradoxus (PP), also **paradoxic pulse**
  and **paradoxical pulse** An exaggeration of the
  normal variation in the pulse during the

inspiratory phase of respiration in which the pulse becomes weaker as one inhales and stronger as one exhales. It is a sign that is indicative of several conditions including cardiac tamponade and lung diseases (e.g., asthma, COPD).

PULSE POINTS

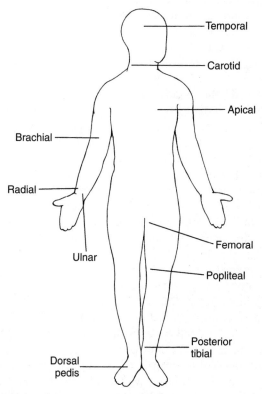

FIGURE 4-1 Pulse points. (From Potter PA, Perry AG, Stockert PA, Hall A: *Fundamentals of nursing*, ed 8, St. Louis, 2013, Mosby.)

RESPIRATION

Normal Ranges

Infant: 30–50 respirations per minute
Child: 20 to 30 respirations per minute
Adult: 12 to 20 respirations per minute

Assessments

Depth Deep or shallow
Rhythm Even or uneven
Effort Ease, quiet, or with great effort
Expansion Symmetric or asymmetric
Cough Productive, nonproductive, or absent
Auscultation Clear, adventitious; crackles, wheezes; diminished, absent, no sounds

Abnormal Patterns of Breathing

Ataxic respiration Irregularity of breathing with irregular pauses and increasing periods of apnea. Caused by damage to the medulla oblongata because of strokes or trauma.

Agonal respiration Characterized by shallow, slow, irregular inspirations followed by irregular pauses. They may also be characterized as gasping or labored breathing accompanied by strange vocalizations. The cause is cerebral ischemia because of extreme hypoxia or even anoxia.

Apneustic respiration Characterized by deep, gasping inspiration with a pause at full inspiration followed by a brief, insufficient release. Caused by damage to the pons or upper medulla from strokes or trauma.

Cheyne–Stokes respiration Characterized by periods of breathing with gradually increasing and decreasing tidal volume. Caused by the failure of the respiratory center.

Biot's respiration or cluster respirations Characterized by groups of quick, shallow inspirations followed by regular or irregular periods of apnea. Caused by damage to the medulla oblongata.

Sleep apnea Characterized by temporary cessation of respiration. Caused by enlarged tonsils or adenoids, extreme obesity, or obstruction of the nasal airway.

Kussmaul breathing Characterized by deep, regular breathing with a rate of fast, normal, or slow. Caused by metabolic acidosis, diabetic acidosis, and coma.

Apnea Characterized by the cessation of respiration lasting from 2 to 60 seconds. Caused by respiratory distress syndrome, bronchopulmonary dysplasia early cessation of theophylline or aminophylline, convulsions, intracranial or subdural hemorrhage, or cerebral edema.

BLOOD PRESSURE
Normal Averages (Systolic/Diastolic)
Newborn: 65–90/30–60 mm Hg
Infant: (1 year) 65–125/40–90 mm Hg
   (2 years) 75–100/40–90 mm Hg
Child: (4 years) 80–120/45–85 mm Hg
   (6 years) 85–115/50–60 mm Hg
Adolescent: (12 years) 95–135/50–70 mm Hg
    (16 years) 100–140/50–70 mm Hg
Adult: (18–60 years) 110–140/60–90 mm Hg
   (60+ years) 120–140/80–90 mm Hg

Orthostatic or Postural Changes
Take blood pressure and pulse with patient lying down. Then have patient sit or stand for 1 minute. Retake blood pressure and pulse. Record both sets of numbers. If patient is orthostatic, pressure will decrease (20–30 mm Hg) and pulse will increase (5–25 beats per minute) when sitting or standing.
 Record and report any orthostasis.

Korotkoff Sounds

Sounds of Blood Pressure

Phase I Systole (sharp thud)

Phase II Systole (swishing sound)

Phase III Systole (low thud or knocking)

Phase IV Diastole (begins fading)

Phase V Diastole (silence)

Blood volume Amount of blood in the system

Decreased blood volume Equals decreased pressure, meaning increased need for fluids

Increased blood volume Equals increased pressure, meaning need for fewer fluids

Cardiac output Stroke volume multiplied by heart rate

Diastole Ventricular relaxation

Pulse pressure Systole minus diastole (normal range is 25–50)

Systole Ventricular contraction

Viscosity Thickness of the blood

Increased viscosity Equals increased pressure, meaning more work on the heart

The Cuff

Cuff should be 20% wider than the diameter of the limb.

Creating a False High Reading

- Having a cuff that is too narrow
- Having a cuff that is too loose
- Deflating the cuff too slowly
- Having the arm below the heart
- Having the arm unsupported

Creating a False Low High Reading

- Having a cuff that is too wide
- Having a cuff that is too tight
- Deflating the cuff too quickly
- Having the arm above the heart

Creating a False Diastolic Reading
- Deflating the cuff too slowly
- Having a stethoscope that fits poorly in the examiner's ears
- Inflating the cuff too slowly

Creating a False Systolic Reading
- Deflating the cuff too quickly

Height and Weight Conversions*			
Height			
Inches	cm	cm	Inches
1	2.5	1	0.4
2	5.1	2	0.8
4	10.2	3	1.2
6	15.2	4	1.6
8	20.3	5	2.0
10	25.4	6	2.4
20	50.8	8	3.1
30	76.2	10	3.9
40	101.6	20	7.9
50	127.0	30	11.8
60	152.4	40	15.7
70	177.8	50	19.7
80	203.2	60	23.6
90	227.6	70	27.6
100	254.0	80	31.5
150	381.0	90	35.4
200	508.0	100	39.4

*1 inch = 2.54 cm; 1 cm = 0.3937 inch.
From Thompson JM, Bowers AC: *Clinical outlines for health assessment*, ed 4, St. Louis, 1997, Mosby.

Height and Weight Conversions*			
Weight			
lb	**kg**	**kg**	**lb**
1	0.5	1	2.2
2	0.9	2	4.4
4	1.8	3	6.6
6	2.7	4	8.8
8	3.6	5	11.0
10	4.5	6	13.2
20	9.1	8	17.6
30	13.6	10	22
40	18.2	20	44
50	22.7	30	66
60	27.3	40	88
70	31.8	50	110
80	36.4	60	132
90	40.9	70	154
100	45.4	80	176
150	66.2	90	198
200	90.8	100	220

*1 lb = 0.454 kg; 1 kg = 2.204 lb.

1983 Metropolitan Height and Weight Tables for Adults*

MEN			Small Frame		Medium Frame		Large Frame	
Feet	Inches	cm	Pounds	Kilograms†	Pounds	Kilograms†	Pounds	Kilograms†
5	1	154.9	128–134	58.2–60.9	131–141	59.5–64.1	138–150	62.7–68.2
5	2	157.5	130–136	59.1–61.8	133–143	60.4–65.0	140–153	63.6–69.5
5	3	160.0	132–138	60.0–62.7	135–145	61.4–65.9	142–156	64.5–70.9
5	4	162.6	134–140	60.9–63.6	137–148	62.3–67.2	144 160	65.5–72.7
5	5	165.1	136–142	61.8–64.5	139–151	63.2–68.6	146–164	66.4–74.5
5	6	167.6	138–145	62.7–65.9	142–154	64.5–70.0	149–168	67.7–76.4
5	7	170.2	140–148	63.6–67.2	145–157	65.9–71.4	152–172	69.1–78.2
5	8	172.7	142–151	64.5–68.6	148–160	67.2–72.7	155–176	70.5–80.0
5	9	175.3	144–154	65.5–70.0	151–163	68.6–74.1	158–180	71.8–81.8
5	10	177.8	146–157	66.4–71.4	154–166	70.0–75.3	161–184	73.2–83.6
5	11	180.3	149–160	67.7–72.7	157–170	71.4–77.3	164–188	74.5–85.5
6	0	182.9	152–164	69.1–74.5	160–174	72.7–79.1	168–192	76.4–87.3
6	1	185.4	155–168	70.5–76.4	164–178	74.5–80.9	172–197	78.2–89.5
6	2	188.0	158–172	71.8–78.2	167–182	75.9–82.7	176–202	80.0–91.8
6	3	190.5	162–176	73.6–80.0	171–187	77.7–85.0	181–207	82.3–94.1

Modified from Metropolitan Life Insurance Company, Statistical Bulletin (source of basic data: *1979 Build Study, Society of Actuaries and Association of Life Insurance Medical Directors of America,* 1980), New York, 1983, Metropolitan Life Insurance Company.

Continued

1983 Metropolitan Height and Weight Tables for Adults—cont'd

WOMEN		Small Frame		Medium Frame		Large Frame	
Feet	Inches	cm	Pounds	Kilograms†	Pounds	Kilograms†	Pounds	Kilograms†
4	9	144.8	102–111	46.4–50.0	109–121	49.5–55.0	118–131	53.6–59.5
4	10	147.3	102–113	46.8–51.4	111–123	50.0–55.9	120–134	54.5–60.9
4	11	149.9	104–115	47.3–52.3	113–126	51.4–57.2	122–137	55.5–62.3
5	0	152.4	106–118	48.2–53.6	115–129	52.3–58.6	125–140	56.8–63.6
5	1	154.9	108–121	49.1–55.0	118–132	53.6–60.0	128–143	58.2–65.0
5	2	157.5	111–124	50.5–56.4	121–135	55.0–61.4	131–147	59.5–66.8
5	3	160.0	114–127	51.8–57.7	124–138	56.4–62.7	134–151	60.9–68.6
5	4	162.6	117–130	53.2–59.0	127–141	57.7–64.1	137–155	62.3–70.5
5	5	165.1	120–133	54.5–60.5	130–144	59.0–65.5	140–159	63.6–72.3
5	6	167.6	123–136	55.9–61.8	133–147	60.5–66.8	143–163	66.0–74.1
5	7	170.2	126–139	57.3–63.2	136–150	61.8–68.2	146–167	66.4–75.9
5	8	172.7	129–142	58.6–64.5	139–153	63.2–69.5	149–170	67.7–77.3
5	9	175.3	132–145	60.0–65.9	142–156	64.6–70.9	152–173	69.1–78.6
5	10	177.8	135–148	61.4–67.3	145–159	65.9–72.3	155–176	70.5–80.0
5	11	180.3	138–151	62.7–73.6	148–162	67.3–73.6	158–179	71.8–81.4

*The weights presented are those associated with the lowest mortality. They are not necessarily the weights at which people are healthiest, perform their jobs optimally, or even look their best. Weights are for persons 25–59 years old (in indoor clothing). Three weight ranges were determined for each sex on each size and attributed to a small, medium, or large frame (in indoor clothing weighing 5 lb for men and 3 lb for women; shoes with 1-inch heels).

†Kilogram ranges determined through direct conversion of pound ranges (# of lb ÷ 2.2 = # of kg).

CHAPTER 5

Documentation

For an in-depth study of documentation, consult the
following publications:

Balzer-Riley J: *Communication in nursing: communicating assertively and responsibly in nursing*, ed 7, St. Louis, 2012, Mosby.

Nugent P, Green J, Hellmer Sau MA, Pelikan P: *Mosby's comprehensive review of nursing for the NCLEX-RN examination*, ed 20, St. Louis, 2012, Mosby.

Potter PA, Perry AG, Stockert PA, Hall A: *Fundamentals of nursing*, ed 8, St. Louis, 2013, Mosby.

THE NURSING PROCESS

Assessment Data collection; tools used include patient and family interviews, functional areas, physical assessments, and laboratory tests; subjective aspects are those observed by patient; objective aspects are those observed by nurse

Analysis Interpretation of collected patient data: determination of nursing diagnosis and plan of care; formation of nursing diagnoses

Planning Formation of patient's plan of care; patient goals are outcomes to be achieved by patient

Implementation Nursing interventions; patient's plan of care is based on assessments, analysis, and expected outcomes

Evaluation Degree to which patient's outcomes have been achieved; revision is an alteration in plan of care when expected outcomes are not achieved

EFFECTIVE DOCUMENTATION

Be factual.
Be accurate.
Be complete.
Be concise.
Be current.
Be organized.

DOCUMENTATION OF GOALS AND OUTCOMES

Patient centered Should reflect the patient behavior and responses to nursing interventions

Singular Should address only one behavior or response

Observable Must be able to observe if change takes place in a patient's status

Measurable Should measure the patient's response to nursing care; terms describing quality, quantity, frequency, length, or weight allow you to evaluate outcomes precisely

Time limited Time frames assist in determining if the patient is making progress and promote accountability in the delivery and management of nursing care

Mutual Increases the patient's motivation and cooperation

Realistic Provide patients a sense of hope that increases motivation and cooperation

---

Adapted from Potter PA, Perry AG, Stockert PA, Hall A: *Fundamentals of nursing,* ed 8, St. Louis, 2013, Mosby.

NURSING DIAGNOSES BY FUNCTIONAL AREA
Domain 1: Health Promotion
Class 1: Health Awareness
Deficient Diversional Activity
Sedentary Lifestyle

Class 2: Health Management
Deficient Community Health
Risk-Prone Health Behavior
Ineffective Health Maintenance
Readiness for Enhanced Immunization Status
Ineffective Protection
Ineffective Self-Health Management
Readiness for Enhanced Self-Health Management
Ineffective Family Therapeutic Regimen
    Management

Domain 2: Nutrition
Class 1: Ingestion
Insufficient Breast Milk
Ineffective Infant Feeding Pattern

Imbalanced Nutrition: Less Than Body
   Requirements
Imbalanced Nutrition: More Than Body
   Requirements
Readiness for Enhanced Nutrition
Risk for Imbalanced Nutrition: More Than Body
   Requirements
Impaired Swallowing

Class 2: Digestion
Class 3: Absorption
Class 4: Metabolism
Risk for Unstable Blood Glucose Level
Neonatal Jaundice
Risk for Neonatal Jaundice
Risk for Impaired Liver Function

Class 5: Hydration
Risk for Electrolyte Imbalance
Readiness for Enhanced Fluid Balance
Deficient Fluid Volume
Excess Fluid Volume
Risk for Deficient Fluid Volume
Risk for Imbalanced Fluid Volume

Domain 3: Elimination and Exchange
Class 1: Urinary Function
Functional Urinary Incontinence
Overflow Urinary Incontinence
Reflex Urinary Incontinence
Stress Urinary Incontinence
Urge Urinary Incontinence
Risk for Urge Urinary Incontinence
Impaired Urinary Elimination
Readiness for Enhanced Urinary Elimination
Urinary Retention

Class 2: Gastrointestinal Function
Constipation
Perceived Constipation
Risk for Constipation
Diarrhea
Dysfunctional Gastrointestinal Motility
Risk for Dysfunctional Gastrointestinal Motility
Bowel Incontinence

Class 3: Integumentary Function
Class 4: Respiratory Function
Impaired Gas Exchange

Domain 4: Activity/Rest
Class 1: Sleep/Rest
Insomnia
Sleep Deprivation
Readiness for Enhanced Sleep
Disturbed Sleep Pattern

Class 2: Activity/Exercise
Risk for Disuse Syndrome
Impaired Bed Mobility
Impaired Physical Mobility
Impaired Wheelchair Mobility
Impaired Transfer Ability
Impaired Walking

Class 3: Energy Balance
Disturbed Energy Field
Fatigue
Wandering

Class 4: Cardiovascular/Pulmonary Responses
Activity Intolerance
Risk for Activity Intolerance
Ineffective Breathing Pattern

Decreased Cardiac Output
Risk for Ineffective Gastrointestinal Perfusion
Risk for Ineffective Renal Perfusion
Impaired Spontaneous Ventilation
Ineffective Peripheral Tissue Perfusion
Risk for Decreased Cardiac Tissue Perfusion
Risk for Ineffective Cerebral Tissue Perfusion
Risk for Ineffective Peripheral Tissue Perfusion
Dysfunctional Ventilatory Weaning Response

Class 5: Self-Care
Impaired Home Maintenance
Readiness for Enhanced Self-Care
Bathing Self-Care Deficit
Dressing Self-Care Deficit
Feeding Self-Care Deficit
Toileting Self-Care Deficit
Self-Neglect

Domain 5: Perception/Cognition
Class 1: Attention
Unilateral Neglect

Class 2: Orientation
Impaired Environmental Interpretation
    Syndrome

Class 3: Sensation/Perception
Class 4: Cognition
Acute Confusion
Chronic Confusion
Risk for Acute Confusion
Ineffective Impulse Control
Deficient Knowledge
Readiness for Enhanced Knowledge
Impaired Memory

Class 5: Communication
Readiness for Enhanced Communication
Impaired Verbal Communication

Domain 6: Self-Perception
Class 1: Self-Concept
Hopelessness
Risk for Compromised Human Dignity
Risk for Loneliness
Disturbed Personal Identity
Risk for Disturbed Personal Identity
Readiness for Enhanced Self-Concept

Class 2: Self-Esteem
Chronic Low Self-Esteem
Situational Low Self-Esteem
Risk for Chronic Low Self-Esteem
Risk for Situational Low Self-Esteem

Class 3: Body Image
Disturbed Body Image

Domain 7: Role Relationships
Class 1: Caregiving Roles
Ineffective Breastfeeding
Interrupted Breastfeeding
Readiness for Enhanced Breastfeeding
Caregiver Role Strain
Risk for Caregiver Role Strain
Impaired Parenting
Readiness for Enhanced Parenting
Risk for Impaired Parenting

Class 2: Family Relationships
Risk for Impaired Attachment
Dysfunctional Family Processes

Interrupted Family Processes
Readiness for Enhanced Family Processes

Class 3: Role Performance
Ineffective Relationship
Readiness for Enhanced Relationship
Risk for Ineffective Relationship
Parental Role Conflict
Ineffective Role Performance
Impaired Social Interaction

Domain 8: Sexuality
Class 1: Sexual Identity
Class 2: Sexual Function
Sexual Dysfunction
Ineffective Sexuality Pattern

Class 3: Reproduction
Ineffective Childbearing Process
Readiness for Enhanced Childbearing Process
Risk for Ineffective Childbearing Process
Risk for Disturbed Maternal–Fetal Dyad

Domain 9: Coping/Stress Tolerance
Class 1: Post-Trauma Responses
Post-Trauma Syndrome
Risk for Post-Trauma Syndrome
Rape-Trauma Syndrome
Relocation Stress Syndrome
Risk for Relocation Stress Syndrome

Class 2: Coping Responses
Ineffective Activity Planning
Risk for Ineffective Activity Planning
Anxiety
Defensive Coping
Ineffective Coping

Readiness for Enhanced Coping
Ineffective Community Coping
Readiness for Enhanced Community Coping
Compromised Family Coping
Disabled Family Coping
Readiness for Enhanced Family Coping
Death Anxiety
Ineffective Denial
Adult Failure to Thrive
Fear
Grieving
Complicated Grieving
Risk for Complicated Grieving
Readiness for Enhanced Power
Powerlessness
Risk for Powerlessness
Impaired Individual Resilience
Readiness for Enhanced Resilience
Risk for Compromised Resilience
Chronic Sorrow
Stress Overload

Class 3: Neurobehavioral Stress
Autonomic Dysreflexia
Risk for Autonomic Dysreflexia
Disorganized Infant Behavior
Readiness for Enhanced Organized Infant
    Behavior
Risk for Disorganized Infant Behavior
Decreased Intracranial Adaptive Capacity

Domain 10: Life Principles
Class 1: Values
Readiness for Enhanced Hope

Class 2: Beliefs
Readiness for Enhanced Spiritual Well-Being

Class 3: Value/Belief/Action Congruence
Readiness for Enhanced Decision-Making
Decisional Conflict
Moral Distress
Noncompliance
Impaired Religiosity
Readiness for Enhanced Religiosity
Risk for Impaired Religiosity
Spiritual Distress
Risk for Spiritual Distress

Domain 11: Safety/Protection
Class 1: Infection
Risk for Infection

Class 2: Physical Injury
Ineffective Airway Clearance
Risk for Aspiration
Risk for Bleeding
Impaired Dentition
Risk for Dry Eye
Risk for Falls
Risk for Injury
Impaired Oral Mucous Membrane
Risk for Perioperative Positioning Injury
Risk for Peripheral Neurovascular Dysfunction
Risk for Shock
Impaired Skin Integrity
Risk for Impaired Skin Integrity
Risk for Sudden Infant Death Syndrome
Risk for Suffocation
Delayed Surgical Recovery
Risk for Thermal Injury
Impaired Tissue Integrity
Risk for Trauma
Risk for Vascular Trauma

Class 3: Violence
Risk for Other-Directed Violence
Risk for Self-Directed Violence
Self-Mutilation
Risk for Self-Mutilation
Risk for Suicide

Class 4: Environmental Hazards
Contamination
Risk for Contamination
Risk for Poisoning

Class 5: Defensive Processes
Risk for Adverse Reaction to Iodinated Contrast
    Media
Latex Allergy Response
Risk for Allergy Response
Risk for Latex Allergy Response

Class 6: Thermoregulation
Risk for Imbalanced Body Temperature
Hyperthermia
Hypothermia
Ineffective Thermoregulation

Domain 12: Comfort
Class 1: Physical Comfort
Class 2: Environmental Comfort
Class 3: Social Comfort
Impaired Comfort
Readiness for Enhanced Comfort
Nausea
Acute Pain
Chronic Pain
Social Isolation

Domain 13: Growth/Development
Class 1: Growth
Risk for Disproportionate Growth

Class 2: Development
Delayed Growth and Development
Risk for Delayed Development

To make safe and effective judgments using NANDA-I nursing
diagnoses, it is essential that nurses refer to the definitions and
defining characteristics of the diagnoses listed in the work.
Nursing Diagnoses—Definitions and Classification 2012-2014.
Copyright © 2012, 1994–2012 by NANDA International. Used
by arrangement with Blackwell Publishing Limited, a company
of John Wiley & Sons, Inc.

DEVELOPING A PATIENT'S PLAN OF CARE
The components of the patient's plan of care are
based on the nursing process, beginning with the
patient history and assessment. The assessment
information is the basis for developing the nursing
diagnosis. The patient outcomes or intended results
are formed to give direction to the nursing
interventions. The nursing interventions are the
actions needed to achieve the desired patient
outcomes. The four parts of a care plan are shown
on p. 118.

INDIVIDUALIZING CARE PLANS
When a patient care plan is developed, the
following considerations are needed to individualize
the plan to meet each patient's needs:
- Age
- Gender

- Level of education
- Developmental level
- General health status (current and before illness)
- Disabilities (physical or mental)
- Strength
- Support systems
- Cultural background
- Spiritual background
- Emotional status

Patient's Plan of Care			
Nursing Diagnosis	Patient Outcome	Nursing Intervention	Evaluation
The Nursing Diagnosis			
List the diagnosis →	List the goals	→ List the interventions	—
Related to			
Specific problem →	Each action should have an outcome	→ Actions per nurse	Can the patient accomplish the goals?
Secondary to			
Medical diagnosis →	Consider the time needed to achieve the goals	→ Actions per patient	Did the patient accomplish the goals?
As Manifested by			
List the signs and symptoms →	Consider individualizing the care plan	→ Individualize interventions	Did the symptoms resolve?

CRITICAL PATHWAYS

Critical pathways incorporate a multidisciplinary approach to patient care. When developing a patient's plan of care through the use of critical pathways, consider some of the following questions:

Medicine

Which medical treatments will be recommended? How will these treatments affect the plan of care and the patient's outcomes? How will the prognosis affect the plan of care and the patient's outcomes?

Pharmacy

What medications will be prescribed? How will the medications affect the plan of care and the patient's outcomes?

Therapy

Will physical or occupational therapy be prescribed? How will therapy affect the plan of care and the patient's outcomes? What kind of discharge planning is needed? When in the patient's course of treatment should discharge planning begin? How will the discharge plans affect the plan of care and the patient's outcomes?

Social Work

Will financial, social, or family services be needed for the patient? How will these services affect the plan of care and the patient's outcomes?

Chaplain

Will emotional or spiritual support be needed for the patient? How will this support affect the plan of care and the patient's outcomes?

CHARTING

Source-oriented records Include admission sheet, physicians' orders, history, nurses' notes, tests, and reports

Problem-oriented records Include database, problem list, physicians' orders, care plans, and progress notes

Progress Notes

SOAP **S**ubjective data, **o**bjective data, **a**ssessment, **p**lan

SOAPIE **S**ubjective, **o**bjective, **a**ssessment, **p**lan, **i**ntervention, **e**valuation

AIR **A**ssessment, **i**ntervention, **r**esults

PIE **P**lan, **i**ntervention, **e**valuation

DAR Data, action, response

Narrative Notes written in paragraph form

Flowsheet Notes written in graph or checklist

The Patient's Chart is a Legal Document (Paper Chart)

- Be complete, concise, legible, and accurate.
- Use ink, sign all charting, cross out errors with a single line, and initial.
- Do not erase or use correction fluid.
- Do not leave spaces.
- Use standard abbreviations and proper medical terminology.
- Include date and time.
- Use proper grammar and accurate spelling.
- Documentation can be called as evidence in a legal action.
- Do not place a facilities incident report in the patient's chart.

Electronic Medical Record (EMR)

- Is a legal document and can be called as evidence in a legal action.

- Document using ONLY your username and password.
- Do NOT document using someone else's username.
- Double check to ensure that documentation appears in the correct EMR.
- Use standard abbreviations and proper terminology.
- Use proper grammar and accurate spelling.
- Know the organizational policies for releasing information.
- Follow organizational policy for electronic signatures.
- Follow all organizational confidentiality policy regarding the EMR.

According to HIPAA (Health Insurance Portability and Accountability Act), the patient owns the information contained within the EMR and has a right to view the originals and to obtain copies under law. Health care workers need to know and follow the organizational policies for releasing information to patients.

CHANGE-OF-SHIFT REPORT
Includes:
Patient's name, age, room number, and diagnosis
Reason for admission, date, and type of surgery, if applicable
Significant changes during the past 24 hours
Tests and procedures during the previous shift
Tests and procedures for the upcoming shift
Important laboratory data, current physical and emotional assessments

Vital signs if abnormal, intake and output, IV fluid
    status
Activity, discharge planning
Updated changes or effectiveness of care plan on
    appropriate document

CHAPTER 6

Integumentary System

For an in-depth study of the integumentary system, consult the following publications:

Lewis SM, et al: *Medical-surgical nursing*, ed 8, St. Louis, 2011, Mosby.

Nugent P, Green J, Hellmer Saul MA, Pelikan P: *Mosby's comprehensive review of nursing for the NCLEX-RN examination*, ed 20, St. Louis, 2012, Mosby.

Patton K, Thibodeau G: *Structure and function of the human body*, ed 14, St. Louis, 2012, Mosby.

Potter PA, Perry AG, Stockert PA, Hall A: *Fundamentals of nursing*, ed 8, St. Louis, 2013, Mosby.

Weilitz P, Potter PA: *Pocket guide for health assessment*, ed 6, St. Louis, 2007, Mosby.

Common Integumentary Abnormalities

Type	Characteristics	Assess for
Edema	Fluid accumulation	Trauma, murmur, third heart sound
Diaphoresis	Sweating	Pain, fever, anxiety, insulin reaction
Bromhidrosis	Foul perspiration	Infection, poor hygiene
Hirsutism	Hair growth	Adrenal function
Petechiae	Red or purple spots	Hepatic function, drug reactions
Alopecia	Hair loss	Hypopituitarism, medications, fever, starvation

Common Skin Color Abnormalities

Type	Characteristics
Albinism	Decreased pigmentation
Vitiligo	White patches on exposed areas
Mongolian spots	Black and blue spots on back and buttocks
Jaundice	Yellow pigmentation of skin or sclera
Ecchymosis	Black and blue marks; assess for trauma, bleeding time, or hepatic function
Cyanosis	Bluish color of lips, earlobes, or nails; assess lung and heart status

ABNORMALITIES OF THE NAIL BED

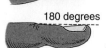

160 degrees

Normal nail: Approximately 160-degree angle between nail plate and nail

180 degrees

Clubbing: Change in angle between nail and nail base (eventually larger than 180 degrees); nail bed softening, with nail flattening; often enlargement of fingertips
Causes: Chronic lack of oxygen: heart or pulmonary disease

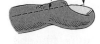

>180 degrees

Beau's lines: Transverse depression in nails indicating temporary disturbance of nail growth (nail grows out over several months)
Causes: Systemic illness such as severe infection, nail injury

Koilonychia (spoon nail): Concave curves
Causes: Iron deficiency anemia, syphilis, use of strong detergents

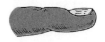

Splinter hemorrhages: Red or brown linear streaks in nail bed
Causes: Minor trauma, subacute bacterial endocarditis, trichinosis

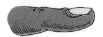

Paronychia: Inflammation of skin at base of nail
Causes: Local infection, trauma

FIGURE 6-1 Abnormalities of nail bed. (From Potter PA, Perry AG, Stockert PA, Hall A: *Fundamentals of nursing*, ed 8, St. Louis, 2013, Mosby.)

Text continued on p. 130

Primary Skin Lesions		
Type	**Definition**	**Example**
Macule	Flat, nonpalpable	Freckle, measles
Papule	Palpable, less than 1 cm diameter	Wart, psoriasis
Vesicle	Palpable, less than 1 cm, with fluid	Blister, chickenpox
Nodule	Hard, less than 1 cm, into dermis	Dermofibroma
Plaque	Palpable or not, greater than 1 cm	Psoriasis, candidiasis
Bulla	Vesicle, greater than 1 cm	Poison oak, impetigo
Tumor	Nodule, greater than 1 cm	Lipoma, fibroma
Pustule	Pus-filled vesicle	Acne
Wheal	Irregular, flat-topped	—
Cyst	Fluid-filled, large	—

Secondary Skin Lesions		
Type	**Definition**	**Example**
Scale	Dead epithelium	Psoriasis
Erosion	Absence of epidermis	Chancre
Crust	Dried exudate	Blister
Fissure	Crack in the epidermis	Cracked lips
Ulcer	Necrotic epidermis	Open sore
Scar	Connective tissue	Healing site
Keloid	Overgrowth of scar	—
Lichenification	Thickening of skin	Eczema
Hyperkeratosis	Thickening of skin	Callus

PRESSURE POINTS

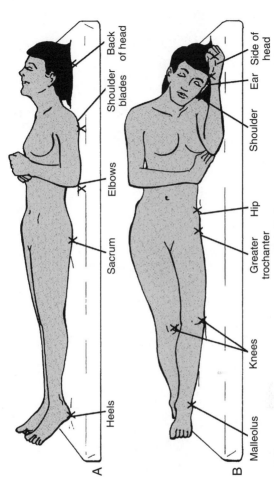

FIGURE 6-2 Pressure points. **A,** Supine position. **B,** Lateral position. (A–E from Sorrentino SA: *Mosby's essentials for nursing assistants,* ed 4, St. Louis, 2010, Mosby.)

Continued

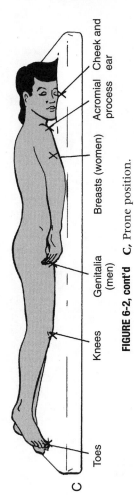

Cheek and ear

Acromial process

Breasts (women)

Genitalia (men)

Knees

Toes

FIGURE 6-2, cont'd **C,** Prone position.

C

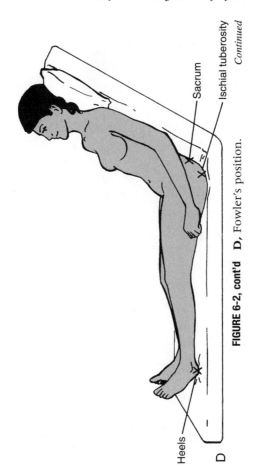

Sacrum

Ischial tuberosity

Heels

Continued

FIGURE 6-2, cont'd D, Fowler's position.

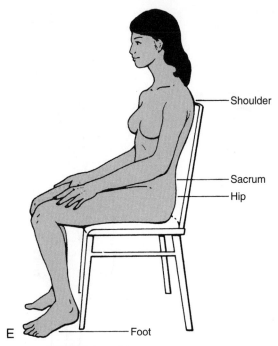

FIGURE 6-2, cont'd   **E,** Sitting position.

PRESSURE ULCER STAGES

In February 2007, the National Pressure Ulcer
Advisory Panel (NPAUP) redefined the stages of
pressure ulcers.

Suspected deep tissue injury: Purplish localized
area of intact skin or blood-filled blister. The
area may be preceded by tissue that is painful,
firm, mushy, boggy, warmer, or cooler compared
with adjacent tissue. Deep tissue injury may be
difficult to detect in individuals with dark skin
tones.

Stage I Intact with nonblanchable redness of a
  localized area usually over a bony prominence.
  Darkly pigmented skin may not have visible
  blanching; its color may differ from the
  surrounding area. The area may be painful, firm,
  soft, warmer, or cooler compared with adjacent
  tissue.

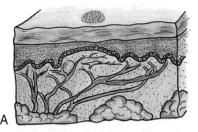

A

FIGURE 6-3 Pressure ulcer stages. **A,** Stage I. (From Potter
PA, Perry, AG, Stockert PA, Hall A: *Basic nursing*, ed 7, St.
Louis, 2011, Mosby.)

Stage II Partial-thickness loss of dermis presenting
  as a shallow open ulcer with a red pink wound
  bed without slough. May also present as an
  intact or open or ruptured serum-filled blister.
  Presents as a shiny or dry shallow ulcer without
  slough or bruising. This stage should not be used
  to describe skin tears, tape burns, perineal
  dermatitis, maceration, or excoriation.

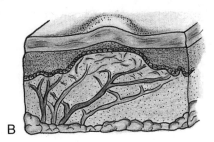

Stage III Full-thickness tissue loss. Subcutaneous fat may be visible, but bone, tendon, and muscle are not exposed. Slough may be present but does not obscure the depth of tissue loss. May include undermining and tunneling.

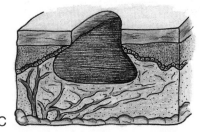

FIGURE 6-3, cont'd   Pressure ulcer stages. **B,** Stage II. **C,** Stage III. (From Potter PA, Perry AG, Stockert PA, Hall A: *Basic nursing*, ed 7, St. Louis, 2011, Mosby.)

Stage IV Full-thickness tissue loss with exposed bone, tendon, or muscle. Slough or eschar may be present on some parts of the wound bed. Often include undermining and tunneling. The depth of a stage IV pressure ulcer varies by anatomical location. Exposed bone or tendon is visible or directly palpable.

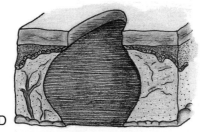

D

FIGURE 6-3, cont'd Pressure ulcer stages. **D,** Stage IV. (From Potter PA, Perry AG, Stockert PA, Hall A: *Basic nursing,* ed 7, St. Louis, 2011, Mosby.)

Unstageable: Full-thickness tissue loss in which the base of the ulcer is covered by slough (yellow, tan, gray, green, or brown) or eschar (tan, brown, or black) in the wound bed. Until enough slough or eschar is removed to expose the base of the wound, the true depth, and therefore stage, cannot be determined. Stable (dry, adherent, intact without erythema, or fluctuance) eschar on the heels serves as "the body's natural (biological) cover" and should not be removed.

The Braden Scale for Predicting Pressure Sore Risk

Patient's Name _____ Evaluator's Name _____ Date of Assessment _____

Sensory Perception

| Ability to respond meaningfully to pressure-related discomfort | 1. Completely limited: Unresponsive (does not moan, flinch, or grasp) to painful stimuli because of diminished level of consciousness or sedation. | 2. Very limited: Responds only to painful stimuli. Cannot communicate discomfort except by moaning or restlessness. | 3. Slightly limited: Responds to verbal commands, but cannot always communicate discomfort or need to be turned. | 4. No impairment: Responds to verbal commands. Has no sensory impairment that would limit ability to feel or voice pain or discomfort. |

	or Limited ability to feel pain over most of body surface.	or Has a sensory impairment that limits the ability to feel pain or discomfort over half of body.	or Has some sensory impairment that limits ability to feel pain or discomfort in one or two extremities.	

Moisture

| Degree to which skin is exposed to moisture | 1. Constantly moist: Skin is kept moist almost constantly by perspiration, urine, and so on. Dampness is detected every time patient is moved or turned. | 2. Very moist: Skin is often, but not always, moist. Linen must be changed at least once a shift. | 3. Occasionally moist: Skin is occasionally moist, requiring an extra linen change approximately once a day. | 4. Rarely moist: Skin is usually dry; linen requires changing only at routine intervals. |

Continued

The Braden Scale for Predicting Pressure Sore Risk—cont'd

Patient's Name _____ Evaluator's Name _____ Date of Assessment _____

		Activity		
Degree of physical activity	1. Bedfast: Confined to bed.	2. Chairfast: Ability to walk severely limited or nonexistent. Cannot bear own weight or must be assisted into chair or wheelchair.	3. Walks occasionally: Walks occasionally during day but for very short distances with or without assistance. Spends majority of shift in bed or chair.	4. Walks frequently: Walks outside the room at least twice a day and is outside of room at least once every 2 hours during waking hours.

Mobility

Ability to change and control body position	1. Completely immobile: Does not make even slight changes in body or extremity position without assistance.	2. Very limited: Makes occasional changes but unable to make frequent or significant changes independently.	3. Slightly limited: Makes frequent although slight changes in position independently.	4. No limitations: Makes major and frequent body changes on position independently.

Continued

The Braden Scale for Predicting Pressure Sore Risk—cont'd			
Patient's Name _____ Evaluator's Name _____ Date of Assessment _____			
Nutrition			
Usual food intake pattern	1. Very poor: Never eats a complete meal. Rarely eats more than a third of food offered. Eats two servings or less of protein, meat, or dairy products per day. Takes fluids poorly. Does not take a liquid dietary supplement.	2. Probably inadequate: Never eats a complete meal. Rarely eats more than half of food offered. Protein intake includes only three servings of meat or dairy products per day. Occasionally takes a dietary supplement.	3. Adequate: Eats over half of meals. Eats a total of four servings of protein each day. Occasionally refuses a meal but takes a supplement.	4. Excellent: Eats most of every meal. Usually eats a total of four or more servings of meat and dairy products. Occasionally eats between meals.

or
Is NPO or maintained on clear liquids or IV lines for more than 5 days.

or
Receives less than optimum amount of liquid diet or tube feeding.

or
Is on tube feeding or TPN regimen that probably meets most of nutritional needs.

The Braden Scale for Predicting Pressure Sore Risk—cont'd

Patient's Name _____ Evaluator's Name _____ Date of Assessment _____

Friction and Shear

1. Problem: Requires moderate to maximum assistance in moving. Complete lifting without sliding against sheets is impossible. Frequently slides down in bed or chair, requiring frequent repositioning with maximum assistance. Spasticity, contractures, or agitation leads to almost constant friction.	2. Potential problem: Moves feebly or requires minimum assistance. During a move, skin probably slides to some extent against sheets, chair, restraints, or other devices. Maintains relatively good position in chair or bed most of the time but occasionally slides down.	3. No apparent problem: Moves in bed and in chair independently and has sufficient muscle strength to lift up completely during move. Maintains good position in bed or chair at all times.

TOTAL SCORE _____

IV, intravenous; NPO, nothing by mouth; TPN, total parenteral nutrition.

	The Mouth	
Structure	Normal	Abnormal	Assess for
Lips	Pinkish	Pallor	Anemia
	Bluish (in black patients)	Pallor	Anemia
	Smooth	Blister	Herpes
	Symmetric	Swelling	Allergic reaction
	Moist	Red, cracked	Vitamin B deficiency
Bucca	Pinkish	Pallor	Anemia, leukoplakia or cancer
	Moist	Blue	Hypoxia
		Dry	Dehydration
Gums	Pinkish	Red, swollen	Phenytoin excess, leukemia, vitamin C deficiency
		Dark lines	Bismuth poisoning

Continued

	The Mouth—cont'd		
Structure	Normal	Abnormal	Assess for
Periodontium	Pinkish	Red, swollen	Calcium deposits
Saliva	Moderate	Excessive	9th or 10th cranial nerve injury
Tongue	Centered	Not centered	12th cranial nerve damage
	Dark pink	Red, sore	Anemia
	Smooth	Decreased papillae	Riboflavin or niacin deficit
	Medium sized	Vertical fissure	Dehydration
		Oversized	Hypothyroidism
Uvula	Centered	Not centered	Tumor
	Moves	Does not move	9th or 10th cranial nerve damage
Tonsils	Pink	Red	Pharyngitis
		Swollen	Tonsillitis

CHAPTER 7

Skeletal System

For an in-depth study of the skeletal system, consult the following publications:

Lewis SM, et al: *Medical-surgical nursing*, ed 8, St. Louis, 2011, Mosby.

Nugent P, Green J, Hellmer Saul MA, Pelikan P: *Mosby's comprehensive review of nursing for the NCLEX-RN examination*, ed 20, St. Louis, 2012, Mosby.

Patton K, Thibodeau G: *Structure and function of the human body*, ed 14, St. Louis, 2012, Mosby.

Potter PA, Perry AG, Stockert PA, Hall A: *Fundamentals of nursing*, ed 8, St. Louis, 2013, Mosby.

Weilitz P, Potter PA: *Pocket guide for health assessment*, ed 6, St. Louis, 2007, Mosby.

SKELETON—ANTERIOR VIEW

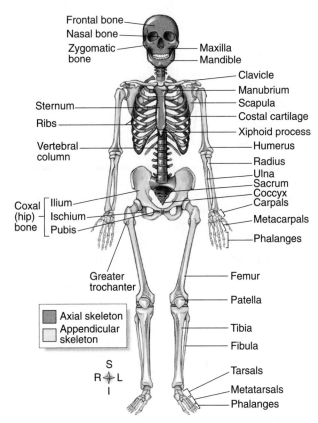

FIGURE 7-1 Skeleton—anterior view. (From Patton K, Thibodeau G: *Structure and function of the human body*, ed 14, St. Louis, 2012, Mosby.)

SKELETON—POSTERIOR VIEW

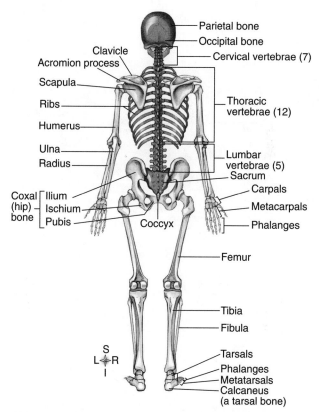

FIGURE 7-2 Skeleton—posterior view. (From Patton K, Thibodeau G: *Structure and function of the human body*, ed 14, St. Louis, 2012, Mosby.)

BONES OF THE SKULL—FRONTAL VIEW

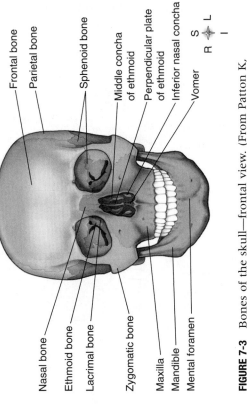

FIGURE 7-3 Bones of the skull—frontal view. (From Patton K, Thibodeau G: *Structure and function of the human body*, ed 14, St. Louis, 2012, Mosby.)

BONES OF THE SKULL—LATERAL VIEW

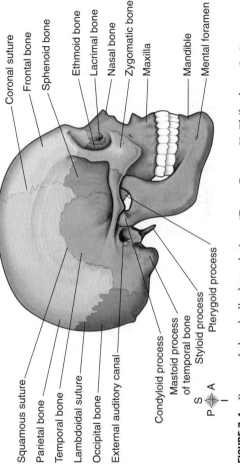

FIGURE 7-4 Bones of the skull—lateral view. (From Patton K, Thibodeau G: *Structure and function of the human body,* ed 14, St. Louis, 2012, Mosby.)

TYPES OF FRACTURES

Closed simple Fracture does not break skin

Comminuted Bone is splintered into fragments

Compression Caused by compressive force; common in lumbar vertebrae

Depressed Broken skull bone driven inward

Displaced Fracture produces fragments that become misaligned

Greenstick Fracture in which one side of bone is broken and other side is bent

Impacted telescoped Bone is broken and wedged into another break

Incomplete Continuity of the bone has not been completely destroyed

Longitudinal Break runs parallel with the bone

Oblique Fracture line runs at a 45-degree angle across the longitudinal axis

Open compound Fracture breaks through skin (can be categorized into grades 1–4 depending on severity)

Pathologic A disease process weakens bone structure so that a slight degree of trauma can cause fracture (most common in osteoporosis and cancers of the bone)

Segmental Fracture in two places (also called *double fracture*)

Silver-fork Fracture of lower end of radius

Spiral Break coils around the bone; can be caused by a twisting force

Transverse Fracture breaks across the bone at a 90-degree angle along the longitudinal axis

Possible Complications from Fractures	
Complication	**Early Clinical Signs**
Pulmonary embolism	Substernal pain, dyspnea, rapid weak pulse; *may occur without symptoms*
Fat embolism	Mental confusion, restlessness, fever, tachycardia, dyspnea
Gas gangrene	Mental aberration, infection
Tetanus	Tonic twitching, difficulty opening mouth; *may occur without symptoms*
Infection	Pain, redness, swelling
Compartment syndrome	Deep localized pain, numbness, weakness Decreased circulation distal to the fracture

TYPES OF TRACTION

Traction is a process in which a steady pull is placed on a part or parts of the body. Traction can be used in reducing a fracture, maintaining a body position, immobilizing a limb, overcoming a muscle spasm, stretching an adhesion, and correcting deformities.

Countertraction A force that pulls against traction

Suspension traction A process to suspend a body part with use of frames, splints, slings, ropes, pulleys, and weights

Skin traction A process of applying wide bands directly to the skin and attaching weights to them; also called Buck's and Russell's

Buck's traction A process of applying a straight pull on the affected extremity; used for muscle spasms and to immobilize a limb

Russell's traction Knee is suspended in a sling to which a rope is attached; allows for some movement and permits flexion of the knee joint; often used with a femur fracture

Skeletal traction A process in which traction is applied directly to the bone; a wire or pin is inserted through the bone distal to the fracture

Bryant's traction (Bryant's extension) Traction applied to the lower leg with the force pulling vertically; used especially in fractures of the femur in infants and young children

Dunlop's traction Used on children with certain fractures of the upper arm when the arm must be kept in a flexed position to prevent problems with the circulation and nerves around the elbow

TYPES OF SYNOVIAL JOINTS

Ball and socket Head of one bone fits into socket of another bone; has greatest range of motion. *Examples:* hip and shoulder

Hinge Convex end of one bone fits into concave end of another bone; movement is on one plane; joints can flex or extend. *Examples:* elbow, knee, ankle, fingers, and toes

Pivot Arch shaped; rotates only. *Examples:* C1 and C2 vertebrae

Saddle Convex bone fits into concave bone; movement is on two planes; joints can flex or extend and abduct or adduct. *Example:* thumb

Gliding Two flat bones move over each other. *Examples:* carpal, tarsal, clavicle, sternum, ribs, vertebrae, fibula, and tibia

Condyloid Oval; circular movement. *Example:* wrist

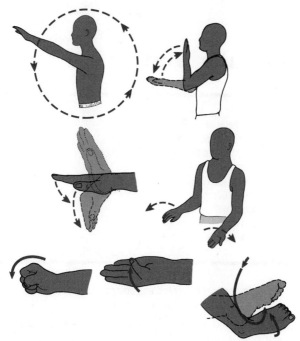

FIGURE 7-5 Types of joints. (Adapted from Potter PA, Perry AG: *Fundamentals of nursing*, ed 7, St. Louis, 2009, Mosby.)

CHAPTER 8

Muscular System

For an in-depth study of the muscular system, consult the following publications:

Lewis SM, et al: *Medical-surgical nursing*, ed 8, St. Louis, 2011, Mosby.
Nugent P, Green J, Hellmer Saul MA, Pelikan P: *Mosby's comprehensive review of nursing for the NCLEX-RN examination*, ed 20, St. Louis, 2012, Mosby.
Patton K, Thibodeau G: *Structure and function of the human body*, ed 14, St. Louis, 2012, Mosby.
Potter PA, Perry AG, Stockert PA, Hall A: *Fundamentals of nursing,* ed 8, St. Louis, 2013, Mosby.
Weilitz P, Potter PA: *Pocket guide for health assessment*, ed 6, St. Louis, 2007, Mosby.

ANTERIOR SUPERFICIAL MUSCLES

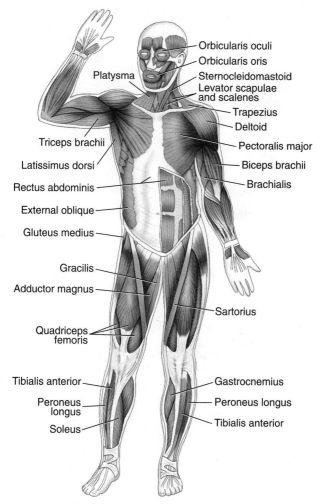

FIGURE 8-1 Anterior superficial muscles.

POSTERIOR SUPERFICIAL MUSCLES

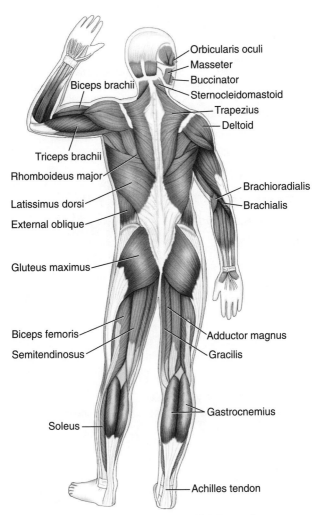

FIGURE 8-2 Posterior superficial muscles.

LATERAL FACIAL MUSCLES

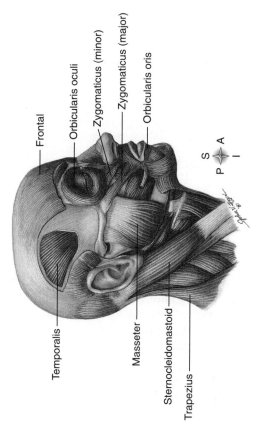

FIGURE 8-3 Lateral facial muscles. (From Patton K, Thibodeau G: *Structure and function of the human body*, ed 14, St. Louis, 2012, Mosby.)

Grading Muscle Strength		
Scale	Percent	Interpretation
5	100	Normal
4	75	Full movement but not against resistance
3	50	Normal movement against gravity
2	25	Movement if gravity eliminated
1	10	No movement
0	0	Paralysis

The "0/5 to 5/5" scale
- 0/5: no contraction
- 1/5: muscle flicker but no movement
- 2/5: movement possible but not against gravity; NOTE: test the joint in its horizontal plane
- 3/5: movement possible against gravity; NOTE: do not test against resistance
- 4/5: movement possible against some resistance; NOTE: this category can be subdivided into 4⁻/5, 4/5, and 4⁺/5
- 5/5: normal strength

EFFECTS OF IMMOBILITY
Benefits
Decreased need for oxygen
Decreased metabolism and energy use
Reduced pain

Bowel Changes
Constipation caused by decreased peristalsis
Poorer sphincter and abdominal muscle tone

Cardiac Changes

Heart rate increase of one-half beat per day caused by increased sympathetic activity

Decreased stroke volume and cardiac output caused by increased heart rate

Hypotension caused by vasodilatation, leading to thrombosis or edema

Integumentary Changes

Decreased turgor caused by fluid shifts

Increased decubitus ulcers caused by prolonged pressure

Increased skin atrophy caused by decreased nutrition

Metabolic Changes

Decreased metabolic rate

Increased catabolism (protein breakdown) leading to a negative nitrogen imbalance, which results in poorer healing

Hypoproteinemia leading to fluid shifts and edema

Musculoskeletal Changes

Decreased muscle strength of 20% per week

Decreased physical endurance and muscle mass

Muscle atrophy caused by decreased contractions

Osteoporosis caused by increased calcium extraction

Demineralization begins on second day of immobilization

Increased fractures caused by porous bones

Increased hypercalcemia

Muscle shortening leading to contracture

Respiratory Changes

Less alveoli expansion caused by less sighing

Increased mucus in lungs caused by less ability to clear them

Decreased chest movement restricts lung expansion
Stiff intercostal muscles caused by less stretching
Shallow respirations leading to decreased capacity
Increased secretions caused by supine position of
  lungs
Less oxygen leading to more carbon dioxide, which
  results in acidosis
Atelectasis caused by decreased blood flow

Neurosensory Changes
Decreased tactile sensation
Increased restlessness, drowsiness, and irritability
Increased confusion and disorientation caused by
  hypercalcemia

Urinary Changes
Poor emptying caused by positioning
Urinary stasis leading to more calcium in kidneys,
  leading to increased renal calculi
Urinary retention and distention caused by poor
  emptying
Incontinence caused by poor muscle tone
Inability to void caused by overstretching of the
  bladder
Infection caused by stasis and alkalinity
Urinary reflux caused by stasis, leading to
  infections

RANGE OF MOTION

Range of Motion (ROM)		
Type	**Function**	**Examples**
Flexion	Decrease angle	Bend elbow or knee, chin down, make fist, bend at waist or wrist, lift leg, bend toes
Extension	Increase angle	Straighten elbow or knee, chin straight, hands open, back, fingers, or toes straight
Hyperextension	Straighten joint beyond limits	Head tilted back, fingers pointed up
Abduction	Move away from midline	Legs or arms away from body, fingers spread apart
Adduction	Move toward midline	Legs together, arms at side, fingers together
Rotation	Move around axis	Circle of head, hand, foot, leg, arm, fingers, toes
Eversion	Turn joint outward	Foot or hand pointed away from the body
Inversion	Turn joint inward	Foot or hand pointed toward the body
Pronation	Move joint down	Palm downward, elbow inward
Supination	Move joint up	Palm upward, elbow outward

Text continued on p. 167

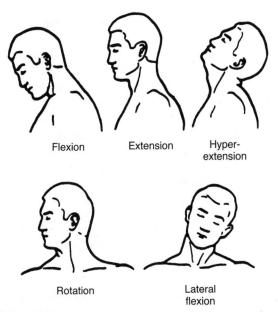

Flexion Extension Hyper-
            extension

Rotation   Lateral
        flexion

FIGURE 8-4 Range-of-motion exercises. (From Monahan F, Sands J, Neighbors M, et al: *Phipps' medical-surgical nursing: health and illness perspectives*, ed 8, St. Louis, 2007, Mosby.)

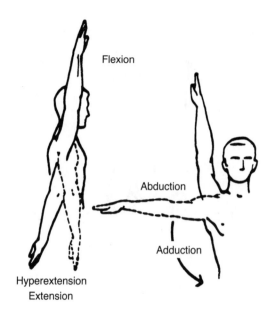

Flexion

Abduction

Adduction

Hyperextension
Extension

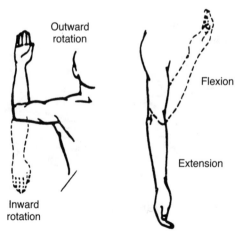

Outward
rotation

Inward
rotation

Flexion

Extension

FIGURE 8-4, cont'd

Continued

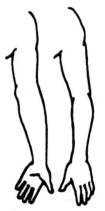

Supination   Pronation

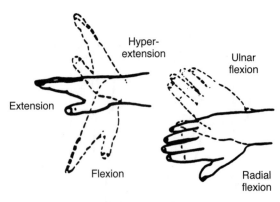

FIGURE 8-4, cont'd

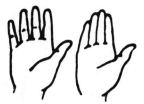

Abduction   Adduction

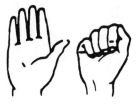

Extension   Flexion

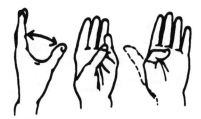

Abduction   Opposition   Extension
Adduction   to little   Flexion
            finger

FIGURE 8-4, cont'd

Continued

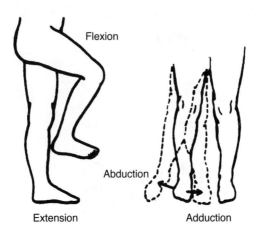

Flexion

Abduction

Extension

Adduction

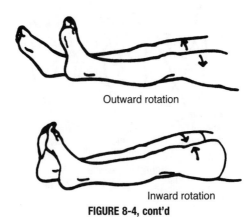

Outward rotation

Inward rotation

FIGURE 8-4, cont'd

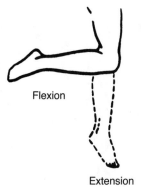

Flexion

Extension
FIGURE 8-4, cont'd
Continued

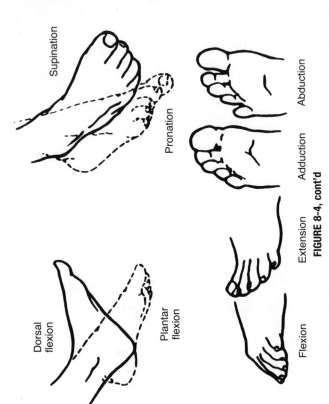

Supination

Pronation

Abduction

Adduction

Dorsal flexion

Plantar flexion

Extension

Flexion

FIGURE 8-4, cont'd

USE OF HEAT*
Local Effects
Increased skin temperature
Vasodilatation, which increases oxygen and
nutrients to area
Increased muscle relaxation
Decreased stiffness and spasm
Increased peristalsis

Indications
Stiffness
Arthritis
Pain

Contraindications
Trauma because of increased bleeding
Edema because of increased fluid retention
Malignant tumors because of increased cell growth
Burns because of increased cell damage
Open wounds because of increased bleeding
Acute areas such as appendix because of possible
rupture
Testes because of destruction of sperm
Sensory-impaired patients because of increased
chance of burns
Confused patients because of increased chance of
injury

USE OF COLD†
Local Effects
Vasoconstriction, which decreases oxygen to area
Decreased metabolism and thus decreased oxygen
needs

---

*The use of heat may require a physician's order but may vary
per facility policy.
†The use of cold may require a physician's order but may vary
per facility policy.

Decreased fluid in area and thus decreased
  swelling
Decreased pain through numbness
Impaired circulation and increased cell death
  caused by lack of oxygen

Indications
Sprains
Fractures
Swelling
Bleeding

Contraindications
Open wounds because of decreased chance of
  healing
Impaired circulation because of increased chance of
  injury
Sensory-impaired patients because of increased
  chance of injury
Confused patients because of increased chance of
  injury

MASSAGE
A Massage Technique

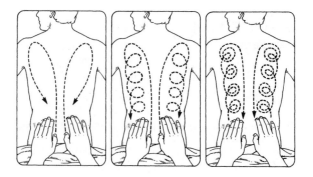

- Assess if massage is contraindicated.
- Start with the patient lying flat or on his or her side.
- Begin with the forehead and work down the body.
- Use a gentle but firm touch.
- Always stroke toward the heart.
- Rub downward on the chest and back.
- Stroke upward on the arms.
- Use a light lotion or oil.

POSITIONING

Dorsal lithotomy Patient lies on back with legs well apart. Knees are bent; stirrups are often used. Position is used to examine the bladder, vagina, rectum, or perineum.

Dorsal recumbent Patient lies on back with legs slightly apart. Knees are slightly bent with the soles of the feet flat on the bed.

Fowler's Patient is partly sitting with knees slightly bent. The head of the bed can be at semi-Fowler's (45 degrees) or high Fowler's (90 degrees).

Knee-chest Patient rests on knees and chest with head turned to the side. Position is used to examine the rectum or vagina.

Left lateral Patient lies on left side with hips closer to the edge of the bed.

Left Sims' Patient lies on left side with right knee bent against abdomen. Used in rectal examinations and giving enemas.

Prone Patient lies on abdomen with arms at sides.

Reverse Trendelenburg Patient lies on back with legs together. Bed is straight with head of bed higher than the foot.

Side lying Patient's head is in straight line with spine. Use pillows to support head, arms, and upper leg.

Supine (horizontal recumbent) Patient lies on back with legs together and extended.

Trendelenburg Patient lies on back with legs together. Bed is straight with head of bed lower than the foot. Used in pelvic surgery.

Positions for Examination

Position	Areas Assessed	Rationale	Limitations
Sitting	Head and neck, back, posterior thorax and lungs, anterior thorax and lungs, breasts, axillae, heart, vital signs, and upper extremities	Sitting upright provides full expansion of lungs and provides better visualization of symmetry of upper body parts.	Physically weakened patient may be unable to sit. Examiner should use supine position with head of bed elevated instead.

Continued

	Positions for Examination—cont'd		
Position	Areas Assessed	Rationale	Limitations
Supine	Head and neck, anterior thorax and lungs, breasts, axillae, heart, abdomen, extremities, pulses	This is the most normally relaxed position. It prevents contracture of abdominal muscles and provides easy access to pulse sites.	If patient becomes short of breath easily, examiner may need to raise head of bed.
Dorsal recumbent	Head and neck, anterior thorax and lungs, breasts, axillae, heart	Patients with painful disorders are more comfortable with knees flexed.	Position is not used for abdominal assessment because it promotes contracture of abdominal muscles.

Position	Image	Body Area	Rationale	Limitations
Lithotomy		Female genitalia and genital tract	This position provides maximal exposure of genitalia and facilitates insertion of vaginal speculum.	Lithotomy position is embarrassing and uncomfortable, so examiner minimizes time that patient spends in it. Patient is kept well draped. Patient with severe arthritis or other joint deformity may be unable to assume this position.
Sims'		Rectum and vagina	Flexion of hip and knee improves exposure of rectal area.	Joint deformities may hinder patient's ability to bend hip and knee.

Continued

Positions for Examination—cont'd

Position	Areas Assessed	Rationale	Limitations
Prone	Musculoskeletal system	This position is used only to assess extension of hip joint.	This position is intolerable for patient with respiratory difficulties.
Knee–chest	Rectum	This position provides maximal exposure of rectal area.	This position is embarrassing and uncomfortable. Patients with arthritis or other joint deformities may be unable to assume this position.

From Potter PA, Perry AG, Stockert PA, Hall A: *Fundamentals of nursing*, ed 8, St. Louis, 2013, Mosby.

CHAPTER 9

Nervous System

For an in-depth study of the nervous system, consult the following publications:

Lewis SM, et al: *Medical-surgical nursing*, ed 8, St. Louis, 2011, Mosby.
Nugent P, Green J, Hellmer Saul MA, Pelikan P: *Mosby's comprehensive review of nursing for the NCLEX-RN examination*, ed 20, St. Louis, 2012, Mosby.

Patton K, Thibodeau G: *Structure and function of the human body*, ed 14, St. Louis, 2012, Mosby.

Potter PA, Perry AG, Stockert PA, Hall A: *Fundamentals of nursing,* ed 8, St. Louis, 2013, Mosby.

Weilitz P, Potter PA: *Pocket guide for health assessment*, ed 6, St. Louis, 2007, Mosby.

STRUCTURES OF THE BRAIN

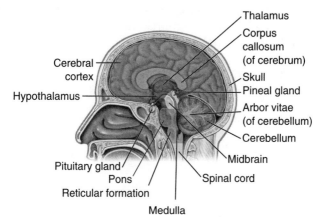

FIGURE 9-1 Structures of the brain. (Modified from Patton K, Thibodeau G: *Structure and function of the human body*, ed 14, St. Louis, 2012, Mosby.)

LEVELS OF CONSCIOUSNESS

Alert Awake and aware, responds appropriately, begins conversation (A&O × 3: alert and oriented to person, place, time)

Lethargic Sleeps but easily aroused, speaks and responds slowly but appropriately

Obtunded Difficult to arouse, slow to respond, and returns to sleep quickly

Stuporous Aroused only through pain, no verbal response, never fully awake

Semicomatose Responds only to pain but has gag and blink reflexes

Comatose No response to pain; no reflexes or muscle tone

NEUROLOGIC FUNCTION

Cerebral
Includes mental status, thought processes, emotions, level of consciousness, orientation, memory language, appropriateness, intelligence, and developmental age

Cranial Nerves
For a summary of the cranial nerves, see p. 189.

Cerebellar
Includes coordination and balance; muscle size, strength, and tone (see p. 190); evaluation of reflexes

Glasgow Coma Scale		Response
Best Eye	Spontaneously	4
Opening	To speech	3
Response	To pain	2
(Record "C" if eyes closed by swelling)	No response	1
Best Motor	Obeys verbal	6
Response to	command	5
Painful Stimuli	Localizes pain	4
(Record best upper limb response)	Flexion—withdrawal	3
	Flexion—abnormal	2
	Extension—abnormal	1
	No response	

Glasgow Coma Scale—cont'd		
Best Verbal		5
Response	Oriented × 3	4
(Record "E" if	Conversation	3
endotracheal	confused	
tube in place;	Speech	2
"T" if	inappropriate	
tracheostomy	Sounds	1
tube in place)	incomprehensible	
	No response	

Modified from Thompson JM, McFarland G, Hirsch J, et al: *Mosby's clinical nursing*, ed 5, St. Louis, 2002, Mosby.

WARNING SIGNS OF IMPENDING STROKE

- Numbness of face, arm, or leg
- Weakness of face, arm, or leg
- Difficult speaking or understanding
- Sudden decreased or blurred vision
- Loss of balance
- Dizziness when accompanied by any of the above signs

Neurologic Deficits by Location		
Location	Possible Deficit	Nursing Interventions
Frontal lobe	Weakness with plegia	Assess function, PT or OT
	Expressive aphasia	Assess for speech therapy
	Focal or grand mal seizures	Educate family on seizures
	Impaired thought, reasoning, and memory; emotional or personality changes	Coordinate neuropsychologic evaluation
Temporal lobe	Visual field loss, impaired memory	Assess visual problems
	Temporal lobe seizures	Monitor for seizures
	Receptive aphasia, dysnomia	Assess speech impairment
Parietal lobe	Sensory deficits, impaired joint position, vibration, light touch	Assess level of neglect
	Impaired left–right discrimination	Refer to PT or OT for assistance
	Sensory seizures, visual field loss	Educate family regarding deficits
		Monitor for seizures

Occipital lobe	Visual hallucinations	Refer to ophthalmologist if needed
	Seizures	Monitor for seizures
		Educate and support family
Cerebellum	Decreased coordination, ataxia	Assess level of deficit
	Nystagmus, increased headaches	Educate and support patient
	Increased intracranial pressure	Monitor headaches
Brainstem	Cranial nerve palsies, ataxia	Assess level of deficit
	Sensory or motor impairment	Safety precautions
	Sudden death	Educate and support family

OT, Occupational therapy; PT, physical therapy.

SEIZURE TERMINOLOGY

Seizure Abnormal electrical activity in the brain

Epilepsy Recurrent unprovoked seizures

Generalized tonic-clonic seizure Previously called *grand mal*. *Tonic* means stiffening, and *clonic* means rhythmic shaking. There is abnormal electrical activity affecting the whole brain (thus the term "generalized").

Partial seizure Sometimes confused with *petit mal*. Only a part of the brain is affected.

Simple partial The patient remains alert and is behaving appropriately.

Complex partial The person is conscious but impaired.

Absence seizure Previously called *petit mal*. This is a generalized seizure *without* shaking.

Postictal state The period after a generalized or partial seizure during which the person usually feels sleepy or confused.

Aura A warning of a seizure. Actually, the aura is an early part of the seizure itself.

Febrile seizures Generally occur in infants and young children; they are most often generalized tonic-clonic seizures. They typically occur in children with a high fever, usually higher than 102°F.

Status epilepticus (SE) A state of continuous or frequently reoccurring seizures lasting 30 minutes or more.

CARE OF THE PATIENT WITH SEIZURES

Equipment and Procedures

Bed should be in the lowest position.

Side rails should be *up* and padded.

Oxygen and suction equipment should be nearby.

Indicate "seizure precautions" on plan of care.

Note if patient has an aura before seizures.
Use digital thermometers, NOT glass thermometers.
Patients should shower rather than use a tub.
Always transport the patient with portable oxygen.
Patients with frequent generalized atonic seizures
    should wear helmets.

During the Seizure
Call for help but DO NOT try to restrain the
    person.
Time the seizure.
STAY WITH THE PERSON.
Help the person to lie down. Place something soft
    under the head.
Turn the person on his or her side if possible.
Remove glasses and loosen tight clothing.
DO NOT place anything between the teeth.
DO NOT attempt to remove dentures.
Monitor the duration of the seizure and the type of
    movement.

After the Seizure
Turn the person to one side to allow saliva to
    drain; suction if needed.
Perform vital signs and neurologic checks as
    needed.
DO NOT offer food or drink until the person is
    fully awake.
Reorient the person.
Notify physician *unless* the person is being
    monitored specifically for seizures.
Notify physician *immediately* if seizure occurs
    without regaining consciousness or if an injury
    occurs.
Record all observations.
Document the time and length of the seizure and if
    there was an aura.

Document the sequence of behaviors during the
  seizures (e.g., eye movement).
Document an injury and what was done about it.
Note what happened with the person just after the
  seizure (did he or she reorient?).

A PATIENT'S SLEEP HISTORY

- Have the patient describe his or her specific
  problem.
- Have the patient describe his or her symptoms
  and alleviating factors.
- Assess the patient's normal sleep pattern.
- Assess the patient's normal bedtime rituals.
- Assess for current or recent physical illnesses.
- Assess for current or recent emotional stress.
- Assess for possible sleep disorders.
- Assess the patient's current medications and
  their possible effects on sleep.

SLEEP DISORDERS

Bruxism Tooth grinding during sleep
Insomnia Chronic difficulty with sleep patterns
   Initial insomnia Difficulty falling asleep
   Intermittent insomnia Difficulty remaining
    asleep
   Terminal insomnia Difficulty going back to
    sleep
Narcolepsy Difficulty in regulating between sleep
  and awake states; person may fall asleep without
  warning
Nocturnal enuresis Bedwetting
Sleep apnea Intermittent periods of cessation of
  breathing during sleep
Sleep deprivation Decrease in the amount and
  quality of sleep
Somnambulism Sleepwalking, night terrors, or
  nightmares

Drugs and Their Adverse Effects on Sleep

Hypnotics
- Interfere with reaching deep sleep stages
- Only temporary increase in quantity of sleep
- May cause "hangover" during day
- Excess drowsiness, confusion, decreased energy
- May worsen sleep apnea in older adults

Diuretics
- Cause nocturia

Antidepressants and Stimulants
- Suppress rapid eye movement (REM) sleep

Alcohol
- Speeds onset of sleep
- Disrupts REM sleep
- Awakens person during night and causes difficulty returning to sleep

Caffeine
- Prevents person from falling asleep
- May cause person to awaken during night

Nonbenzodiazepines
- Anxiety and irritability
- Sleep walking, eating, or driving

Digoxin
- Causes nightmares

Beta-Blockers
- Cause nightmares
- Cause insomnia
- Cause awakening from sleep

Continued

Drugs and Their Adverse Effects on Sleep—cont'd

Valium
- Decreases stages 2 and 4 and REM sleep
- Decreases awakenings

Narcotics (Morphine/Meperidine [Demerol])
- Suppress REM sleep
- If discontinued quickly, can increase risk of cardiac dysrhythmias because of "rebound REM" periods
- Cause increased awakenings and drowsiness

From Potter PA, Perry AG: *Fundamentals of nursing*, ed 7, St Louis, 2009, Mosby.

SEDATION SCALE

S = Sleepy, but easy to arouse
1 = Awake and alert
2 = Slightly drowsy but easy to arouse
3 = Drowsy, drifts to sleep during conversation
4 = Somnolent, minimal or no response to physical stimulation

---

Modified from Pasero C, McCaffery M: *Pain assessment and pharmacological management:* p. 510, St. Louis, 2011, Mosby.

CENTRAL NERVOUS SYSTEM

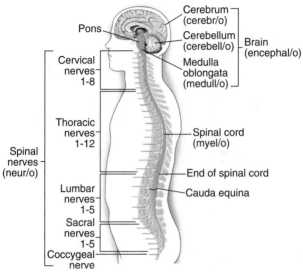

FIGURE 9-2 Central nervous system with spinal nerves.

Assessing Motor Function

Level of Spinal Cord	Assessment: Note Response to the Items Below
C4–C5	Have the patient shrug his or her shoulders against your hands or apply resistance by pushing downward on the patient's shoulders.
C5–C6	Have the patient flex his or her arm at the elbow while you apply resistance by pushing the arm away from the patient.
C7	Have the patient straighten his or her flexed arm and try to keep it flexed while you apply resistance.
	Have the patient pinch his or her thumb and index finger together and hold firmly while you try to pull them apart.
C8–T1	Have the patient squeeze your fingers.
L2–L4	Have the patient lift his or her leg from a lying position while you apply resistance by pushing the leg down.
	Have the patient extend his or her leg from the knee-flexed position while you apply resistance to keep the knee flexed.
L5	Have the patient dorsiflex his or her feet upward while you apply resistance to the dorsal aspects of the feet.
L5–S1	Have the patient bend at the knee while you apply resistance against the move.
S1	Have the patient plantar flex the feet downward while you apply resistance to the plantar aspects of the feet.

Cranial Nerves

Number	Name	Type	Function	Method of Assessment
I	Olfactory	Sensory	Smell	Identify odors
II	Optic	Sensory	Vision	Snellen chart
III	Oculomotor	Motor	Vision	Pupil reaction
IV	Trochlear	Motor	Vision	Vertical vision
		Sensory	Cornea	Blink reflex
V	Trigeminal	Motor	Chewing	Clench teeth
VI	Abducens	Motor	Vision	Lateral vision
VII	Facial	Sensory	Taste	Identify tastes
		Motor	Expression	Smile or frown
VIII	Acoustic	Sensory	Equilibrium	Weber and Rinne tests
IX	Glossopharyngeal	Sensory	Taste	Identify tastes
		Motor	Swallowing	Gag reflex
X	Vagus	Sensory	Pharynx	Identify tastes
		Motor	Vocal	Voice tones
XI	Accessory	Motor	Shoulders	Shrug shoulders
XII	Hypoglossal	Motor	Tongue	Protruding tongue

Types of Reflexes

Name	Elicited by	Proper Response
Babinski	Stroking lateral sole of foot	Great toe fans out
Chaddock	Stroking below lateral malleolus	Great toe fans out
Oppenheim	Stroking tibial surface	Great toe fans out
Gordon	Squeezing calf muscle	Great toe fans out
Hoffmann	Flicking middle finger down	Flexion of the thumb
Ankle clonus	Brisk dorsiflexion of foot with knee flexed	Up and down movement of the foot
Kernig	Straightening leg with thigh muscle flexed	Pain along posterior of thigh
Brudzinski	Flexing chin on chest	Limitations with pain

Reflex Grading Scale

Grade	Symbol	Interpretation
5	5+	Hyperactive (with clonus)
4	4+	Hyperactive (very brisk)
3	3+	Brisk
2	2+	Normal (average)
1	1+	Diminished but present
0	0	Absent

PAIN ASSESSMENT

Gather information about the patient's condition in the following areas.

Definition

The words used by the patient to describe pain, such as *pressure*, *stabbing*, *sharp*, *tingling*, *dull*, *heavy*, or *cold*. It is important to use and understand the patient's language concerning pain and to believe the patient who reports pain.

Onset

When did the pain first begin (date and time)?

Duration

How long does the pain last (persistent, minutes to hours, comes and goes, seconds)? Does the pain occur at the same time each day?

Location

In what area of the body does the pain begin? It may be helpful to have the patient point to the exact area if possible. NOTE: A patient may say the pain is in the stomach but may point over the lower abdominal area. Also ask if the pain radiates, moves, or goes to a different area of the body. Have the patient point to these areas as well.

Severity

How bad is the pain? Or have the patient rate the pain. Have a rating scale ready to use and explain your scale. Use the same scale in subsequent assessments. *Examples:* A 0 to 10 scale with 0 being no pain and 10 being the worst pain or a color scale with blue being no pain and red being the worst pain.

Precipitating Factors
What was the patient doing before the pain began (exercise, bending over, work)?

Aggravating Factors
What makes the pain worse?

Alleviating Factors
What makes the pain get better or go away (pain medications, relaxation, rest, music)?

Associated Factors
Nausea or vomiting?
Anger or agitation?
Depression or drowsiness?
Fatigue or sleeplessness?

Observed Behaviors
Agitation or restlessness?
Bracing or fidgeting?
Rubbing or guarding?
Not eating or sleeping?

Vocalizations
Crying or moaning?
Gasping or groaning?
Sighing or noisy breathing?

Facial Expressions
Grimacing or clenched teeth?
Wincing or furrowed brow?
Sadness or eyes closed?
Frightened or tightened lips?

PAIN RATING SCALES

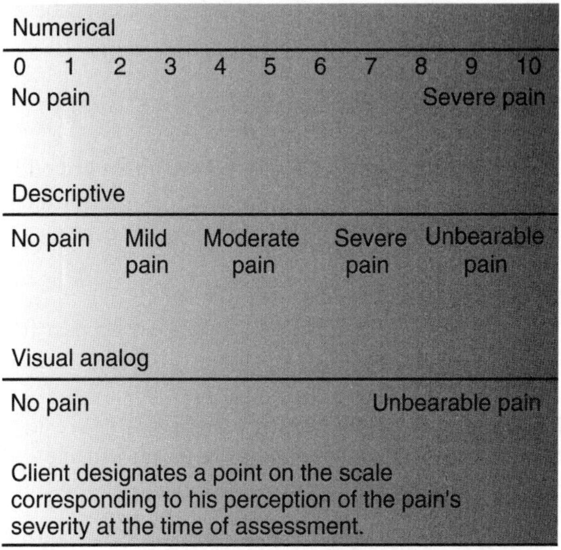

Numerical										
0	1	2	3	4	5	6	7	8	9	10
No pain									Severe pain	

Descriptive				
No pain	Mild pain	Moderate pain	Severe pain	Unbearable pain

Visual analog	
No pain	Unbearable pain

Client designates a point on the scale corresponding to his perception of the pain's severity at the time of assessment.

FIGURE 9-3 Pain rating scales. (From Potter PA, Perry AG, Stockert PA, Hall A: *Fundamentals of nursing,* ed 8, St. Louis, 2013, Mosby.)

NONPHARMACOLOGIC TREATMENTS OF PAIN

Biofeedback Patients can learn to control muscle tension to reduce pain with the use of biofeedback units.

Cold Used to decrease pain or swelling (see p. 167).

Distraction Turning the patient's attention to something other than the pain, such as music, visitors, or scenery.

Heat Used to decrease tension (see p. 167).

Imagery Uses the patient's imagination to create pleasant mental pictures. These pictures are a form of distraction. This activity is said to be a form of self-hypnosis.

Massage See p. 168.

Menthol Used to increase blood circulation to painful areas.

Nerve blocks Used to block severe, unrelieved pain. A local anesthetic, sometimes combined with cortisone, is injected into or around a nerve.

Positioning See pp. 169–174.

Pressure Used to stimulate blood flow to painful areas. Apply firm but not excess pressure for 10 to 60 seconds.

Range of motion exercises See pp. 159–166.

Relaxation Relieves pain by reducing muscle tension. Music or relaxation tapes may be helpful.

TENS (transcutaneous electric nerve stimulation) A mild electric current is thought to interrupt pain impulses.

Vibration Used to simulate blood flow to painful areas.

CHRONIC NONMALIGNANT PAIN: NURSING CARE GUIDELINES*

Do not argue with the patient about whether he or she is in pain.

Do not refer to the patient as a narcotics addict.

Do not tell the patient that he or she will become an addict if he or she continues to receive narcotics.

---

*Modified from McCaffery M, Pasero C: *Pain: clinical manual for nursing practice*, ed 2, St. Louis, 1999, Mosby.

Do not use a placebo to try to determine if the patient has "real" pain.

Be alert to any changes in the patient's pain condition or pain regimen.

Recognize the differences between acute and chronic pain.

Avoid sudden withdrawal of narcotics or sedatives from a patient with chronic pain.

When analgesics are required, give them orally if possible. (The effects of oral analgesics will generally last longer than IV or IM medications.)

Review analgesics being used for relief of chronic versus acute pain.

Offer pain relief alternatives (See pp. 193–194).

Review the patient's support systems and suggest additional ones if appropriate.

Help those living with the patient to understand the patient's pain management routine.

Assess the patient for depression, anxiety, and stress. (Additional stresses may add to the patient's overall pain experience.)

Assess suicidal risk.

	Average Adult Doses for Analgesics			
Drug	**IM Dose (mg/mL)**	**Oral Dose (mg)***	**Half-Life (hr)**	**Duration (hr)**
Aspirin	—	500–1000	15–30 min	4–6
Acetaminophen	—	500–1000	2–3	4–6
Ibuprofen	—	400–800	1.8–2.5	4–6
Salicylate (e.g., Trilisate)	—	500–1000	1–4	6–12
Naproxen	—	500	2–3	6–8
Indomethacin	—	25–75	4–6	8–12
Ketorolac	30–60	10–20	2–3	6
	15–30	—	2–3	6
Celecoxib (Celebrex)	—	200400	8–12	24
Diclofenac (Voltaren)	—	50–200	2–3	4–6
Fenoprofen (Nalfon)	—	200–600	30 min	4–6
Fentanyl	0.05–0.10	Oralet 5 mcg/kg	8 min	1–2
Nabumetone (Relafen)	—	500–750	22–30	—
Piroxicam (Feldene)	—	10–20	30–60	48–72

Oxycodone with acetaminophen (Percocet)	—	5	2–3	4–6
Propoxyphene (Darvon)	—	32–65	1–2	4–6
Levorphanol	2	2–4	2–4	4–8
Morphine	2–15	10–60	1–3	3–7
Codeine	30–60	15–60	2–4	4–6
Hydromorphone (Dilaudid)	1–4	1–10	2–3	4–5
Meperidine (Demerol)	50–100	50–150	1–2	2–4
Methadone	2.5–10	5–40	1–3	4–6
Tramadol (Ultram)	—	50–100	6–8	3–7

*Oral dose, usual dosage range for single dose.

IM, intramuscular.

Data from *Drug facts & comparisons*, St. Louis, 2002, Facts & Comparisons; *Physician's desk reference*, ed 54, Montvale, NJ, 2000, Medical Economics.

THE EYE

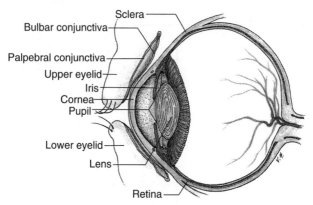

FIGURE 9-4   Structures of the eye. (From Potter PA, Perry AG, Stockert PA, Hall A: *Fundamentals of nursing,* ed 8, St. Louis, 2013, Mosby.)

PUPIL SIZE

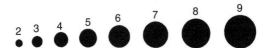

FIGURE 9-5   Chart showing pupil sizes in millimeters. (From Potter PA, Perry AG, Stockert PA, Hall A: *Fundamentals of nursing,* ed 8, St. Louis, 2013, Mosby.)

SIX DIRECTIONS OF GAZE

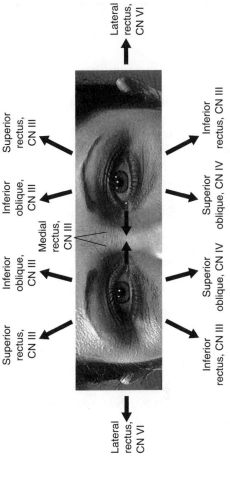

FIGURE 9-6 Directions of gaze. CN = cranial nerve. (From Seidel HM, et al: *Mosby's guide to physical examination*, ed 7, St. Louis, 2011, Mosby.)

Contact Lens Care

Do
- Wash and rinse hands thoroughly before handling a lens.
- Keep fingernails clean and short.
- Remove lenses from the storage case one at a time and place on the eye.
- Start with the same lens (left or right) every time of insertion.
- Use lens placement technique learned from eye specialist.
- Use proper lens care products.
- Wear lenses daily and follow the prescribed wearing schedule.
- Remove a lens if it becomes uncomfortable.
- Keep regular appointments with the eye specialist.
- Remove lenses during sunbathing, showering, and swimming.

Do Not
- Use soaps that contain cream or perfume for cleaning lenses.
- Let fingernails touch lenses.
- Mix up lenses.
- Exceed prescribed wearing time.
- Use saliva to wet lenses.
- Use homemade saline solution or tap water to wet or clean lenses.
- Borrow or mix lens care solution.

Data from Potter PA, Perry AG, Stockert PA, Hall A: *Fundamentals of nursing,* ed 8, St. Louis, 2013, Mosby.

BRAILLE ALPHABET

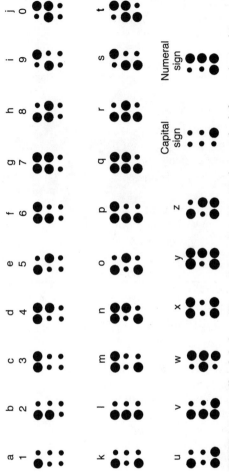

FIGURE 9-7 Braille alphabet. (From Sorrentino SA: *Mosby's textbook for nursing assistants,* ed 7, St. Louis, 2008, Mosby.)

THE EAR

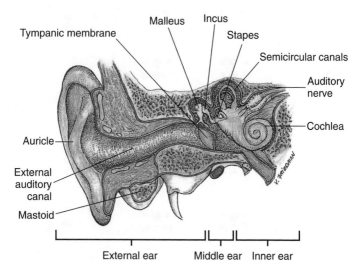

FIGURE 9-8   Structures of the ear. (From Potter PA, Perry AG, Stockert PA, Hall A: *Fundamentals of nursing,* ed 8, St. Louis, 2013, Mosby.)

Assessing Patient's Use of Sensory Aids

Eyeglasses
- Purpose for wearing glasses (e.g., reading distance, or both)
- Methods used to clean glasses
- Presence of symptoms (e.g., blurred vision, photophobia, headaches, irritation)

Contact Lenses
- Type of lenses worn
- Frequency and duration of time lenses are worn (including sleep time)
- Presence of symptoms (e.g., burning, excess tearing, redness, irritation, swelling, sensitivity to light)
- Techniques used by the patient to clean, store, insert, and remove lenses
- Use of eyedrops or ointments
- Use of emergency identification bracelet or card that warns others to remove patient's lenses in case of emergency

Artificial Eye
- Method used to insert and remove eye
- Method for cleaning eye
- Presence of symptoms (e.g., drainage, inflammation, pain involving the orbit)

Hearing Aid
- Type of aid worn
- Methods used to clean aid
- Patient's ability to change battery and adjust hearing-aid volume

From Potter PA, Perry AG: *Fundamentals of nursing,* ed 7, St. Louis, 2009, Mosby.

SIGN LANGUAGE ALPHABET

Manual alphabet

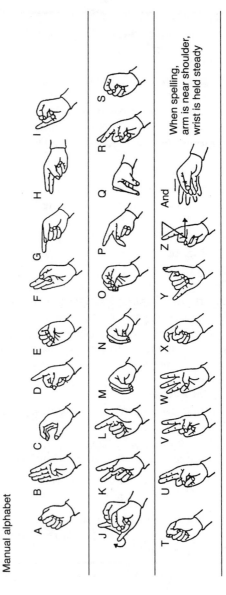

FIGURE 9-9 Sign language alphabet.

SIGN LANGUAGE NUMBERS

Numbers

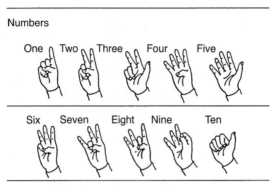

FIGURE 9-10 Sign language numbers.

TIPS FOR COMMUNICATING WITH OLDER ADULTS

- Get the person's attention. This will help if the person is has a hearing impairment.
- Sit face to face. Lip reading may be helpful.
- Appropriate lighting is important. Avoid glare and dimly lit areas.
- Maintain good eye contact. This helps to instill trust.
- Speak slowly and clearly. This helps if the person is hard of hearing.
- Use short, simple words and phrases.
- Ask one question at a time. This may help with sensory overload.
- Give the person extra time to answer. This will help if the person has a hearing impairment.
- Repeat statements or ideas if needed.
- Rephrase, if needed, but do not change the meaning from the first statement.

- Minimize visual and auditory distractions.
- Do not shout. Remember, not everyone is deaf.
- Summarize points if you are not being understood.
- Expect errors or emotional outbursts in a confused person.
- You may need to restart the conversation.
- You may need to stop the conversation if the person is unable to communicate.

CHAPTER 10

Circulatory System

For an in-depth study of the circulatory system, consult the following publications:

Lewis SM, et al: *Medical-surgical nursing*, ed 8, St. Louis, 2011, Mosby.

Nugent P, Green J, Hellmer Saul MA, Pelikan P: *Mosby's comprehensive review of nursing for the NCLEX-RN examination*, ed 20, St. Louis, 2012, Mosby.

Patton K, Thibodeau G: *Structure and function of the human body*, ed 14, St. Louis, 2012, Mosby.

Potter PA, Perry AG, Stockert PA, Hall A: *Fundamentals of nursing*, ed 8, St. Louis, 2013, Mosby.

Weilitz P, Potter PA: *Pocket guide for health assessment*, ed 6, St. Louis, 2007, Mosby.

PRINCIPAL ARTERIES OF THE BODY

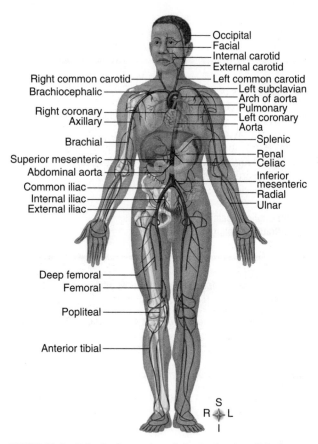

Occipital
Facial
Internal carotid
External carotid
Left common carotid
Left subclavian
Arch of aorta
Pulmonary
Left coronary
Aorta
Splenic
Renal
Celiac
Inferior mesenteric
Radial
Ulnar

Right common carotid
Brachiocephalic
Right coronary
Axillary
Brachial
Superior mesenteric
Abdominal aorta
Common iliac
Internal iliac
External iliac
Deep femoral
Femoral
Popliteal
Anterior tibial

FIGURE 10-1 Principal arteries of the body. (Modified from Patton K, Thibodeau G: *Structure and function of the human body*, ed 14, St. Louis, 2012, Mosby.)

STRUCTURES OF THE HEART

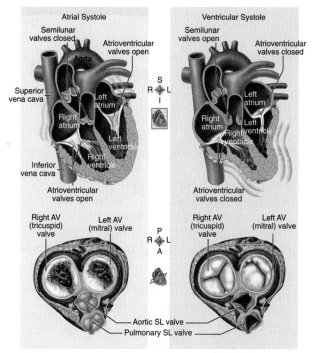

FIGURE 10-2   Structures of the heart. A = anterior; AV = atrioventricular; L = left; P = posterior; R = right; SL = Semi lunar. (Modified from Patton K, Thibodeau G: *Structure and function of the human body*, ed 14, St. Louis, 2012, Mosby.)

CORONARY ARTERIES
Right Coronary Artery
Right atrium arid anterior right ventricle
Supplies blood to:
   Posterior septum (90%)
   Posterior papillary muscle
   Sinus and atrioventricular (AV) nodes
      (80%–90%)
   Inferior aspect of left ventricle

Left Coronary Artery
Left anterior descending (LAD)
Supplies blood to:
   Anterior left ventricular wall
   Anterior papillary muscle
   Left ventricular apex
   Anterior interventricular septum
      Septal branches supply conduction system
      System bundle of His and bundle branches

Circumflex
Supplies blood to:
   Left atrium
   Posterior surfaces of left ventricle
   Posterior aspect of the septum

BASIC CARDIAC ASSESSMENTS
S_1
First heart sound—heard when the mitral and
tricuspid valves close. After ventricles are filled
with blood, a dull, low-pitched "lub" is heard.
Systole begins when ventricles contract. Systole is
shorter than diastole.

S_2
Second heart sound—heard when the aortic and
pulmonic values close. After blood goes to aorta

and pulmonary artery, a high-pitched, snappy "dub" is heard.

CARDIAC HISTORY
Patient History
Heart attacks, rheumatic fever, fevers, hypertension, dizziness, syncope, diabetes, lung or endocrine diseases

Health Habits
Smoking, alcohol, diet, exercise, stress

Family History
Coronary disease, strokes, or obesity in parents or grandparents

Signs and Symptoms
Chest pain, shortness of breath, orthopnea, syncope, hypertension, dyspnea, edema, cough, palpitations, wheezing, need for extra pillow to sleep, fatigue, weakness

TOPOGRAPHIC AREAS FOR CARDIAC AUSCULTATION

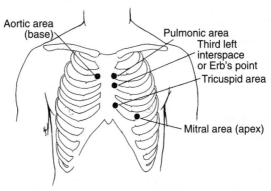

FIGURE 10-3   Topographic areas for cardiac auscultation. (From Monahan F, Sands J, Neighbors M, et al: *Phipps' medical-surgical nursing: health and illness perspectives*, ed 8, St. Louis, 2007, Mosby.)

Location of Maximal Impulse

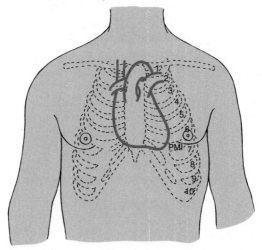

FIGURE 10-4   Location of maximal impulse. (From Potter PA, Perry AG, Stockert PA, Hall A: *Fundamentals of nursing*, ed 8, St. Louis, 2013, Mosby.)

ABNORMAL HEART SOUNDS

S_1 Varying intensity with different beats—indicates possible heart blockage

S_2 Increased intensity at aortic valve—indicates possible hypertension

S_3 Increased intensity at pulmonic valve—indicates possible hypertension

Systole Sharp sound—indicates possible deformity

Diastole Presence of S_3 in elderly adults—indicates possible heart failure

S_1 S_2 S_3 "Ken tuck ky"

S_4 S_1 S_2 "Ten nes see"

Quality and Pitch of Murmurs		
Type	**Quality**	**Pitch**
Aortic and pulmonary stenosis	Harsh	Medium high
Mitral and tricuspid regurgitation	Blowing	High
Ventricular septal defect	Usually harsh	High
Mitral stenosis	Rumbling	Low
Aortic regurgitation	Blowing	High

MURMUR GRADING SCALE

1 Difficult to hear
2 Faint but recognizable
3 Heard easily with stethoscope
4 Loud, often with a palpable thrill
5 Very loud; associated with a thrill
6 Stethoscope not needed to hear; can be heard with stethoscope 1 inch from chest

	Cardiovascular Drugs	
Agent	Side Effects	Consideration
Digoxin (Lanoxin) (IV/PO)	Fatigue, headache, anoxia	Monitor rhythm and blood pressure during administration
Digitoxin (PO)	Arrhythmia, nausea, vomiting	Monitor heart rate and blood pressure
Nitroglycerin (IV, PO, buccal, ointment, transdermal)	Headache, hypotension, nausea, vomiting, flushing, arrhythmia	Monitor for arrhythmia
Amrinone (IV)	Arrhythmia, hypotension, thrombocytopenia	Monitor rhythm, blood pressure, and heart rate
Milrinone (IV)	Arrhythmia, hypotension, thrombocytopenia	Monitor rhythm blood pressure, and heart rate
Dobutamine (IV)	Tachycardia, angina, shortness of breath, headache, ventricular ectopy, nausea	Monitor output Monitor rhythm and blood pressure Check peripheral pulses

Dopamine (IV)	Tachycardia, angina, shortness of breath, headache, ventricular ectopy, nausea	Monitor output Monitor rhythm and blood pressure
Epinephrine (IV)	Arrhythmia, hypertension, headache, hyperglycemia, nausea	Check peripheral pulses Monitor output Monitor rhythm and blood pressure Check peripheral pulses
Norepinephrine	Bradycardia, tachycardia, angina, headache, dizziness	Monitor rhythm and blood pressure Have atropine available Monitor fluid balance
Isoproterenol (IV)	Arrhythmia, hypertension, nausea, vomiting, flushing, headache	Monitor rhythm and blood pressure Monitor for arrhythmia Monitor fluid balance

IV, intravenous; PO, oral.

ASSESSMENT OF PULSE SITES*

Temporal Found over the **temporal bone** above and lateral to the eye; easily accessible, used often in children

Apical Best found between the **fourth and fifth intercostals space,** midclavicular line; used to auscultate heart sounds and before the administration of digoxin

Carotid Found on either side of the neck over the **carotid artery;** used to assess circulation during shock or cardiac arrest and when other peripheral pulses are poor

Brachial Found in the **antecubital area** of the arm; used to auscultate blood pressure and to assess circulation of the lower arm

Radial Found on the **thumb side of the forearm** at the wrist; used to assess circulation of the head and peripheral circulation

Ulnar Found at the **wrist on the opposite side of the radius;** used to assess circulation of the hand and in Allen's assessment test

Femoral Found below the **inguinal ligament** midway between the symphysis pubis and the anterosuperior iliac spine; used to assess circulation of the leg; can be used to assess circulation during shock or cardiac arrest or when other peripheral pulses are poor

Popliteal Found **behind the knee;** used to assess lower leg circulation

Posterior tibial Found on the inner side of each **ankle;** used to assess foot circulation

Dorsalis pedis Found along the **top of the foot** between extension tendons of the great and first toes; used to assess the circulation of the foot

---

*See Figure 4-1, p. 97.

EDEMA GRADING SCALE
1+ Barely detectable
2+ Indentation of less than 5 mm
3+ Indentation of 5 to 10 mm
4+ Indentation of greater than 10 mm

PULSE GRADING SCALE

4-Point Scale		3-Point Scale	
0	Absent	0	Absent
1+	Diminished/Barely palpable	1+	Weak, thready
2+	Normal/Expected	2+	Normal
3+	Full/Strong	3+	Full, bounding
4+	Bounding		

Tissue Perfusion		
Area	**Abnormality**	**Reveals**
Skin color	Cyanotic	Decreased venous return
	Pallor	Decreased arterial flow
	Dusky	Decreased arterial flow
Temperature	Cool	Decreased arterial flow
Fluid	Mild edema	Decreased arterial flow
	Great edema	Decreased venous return
Texture	Thin or thick	Decreased venous return and arterial flow
	Shiny	Decreased venous return and arterial flow
Nails	Cyanotic	Decreased arterial flow

CHAPTER 11

Respiratory System

For an in-depth study of the respiratory system,
consult the following publications:

Lewis SM, et al: *Medical-surgical nursing*, ed 8, St. Louis, 2011, Mosby.
Nugent P, Green J, Hellmer Saul MA, Pelikan P: *Mosby's comprehensive review of nursing for the NCLEX-RN examination*, ed 20, St. Louis, 2012, Mosby.
Patton K, Thibodeau G: *Structure and function of the human body*, ed 14, St. Louis, 2012, Mosby.
Potter PA, Perry AG, Stockert PA, Hall A: *Fundamentals of nursing,* ed 8, St. Louis, 2013, Mosby.
Weilitz P, Potter PA: *Pocket guide for health assessment*, ed 6, St. Louis, 2007, Mosby.

STRUCTURES OF THE RESPIRATORY TRACT

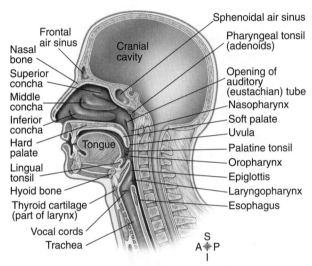

FIGURE 11-1 Upper respiratory tract. (Modified from Thibodeau G, Patton K: *Structure and function of the human body*, ed 14, St. Louis, 2012, Mosby.)

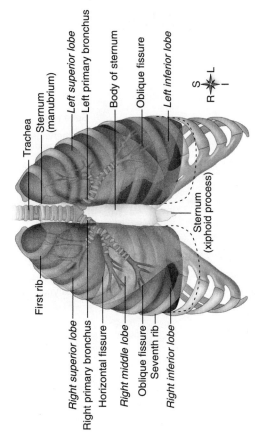

FIGURE 11-2 Structures of the lungs. (Modified from Thibodeau G, Patton K: *Structure and function of the human body*, ed 14, St. Louis, 2012, Mosby.)

CHEST WALL LANDMARKS

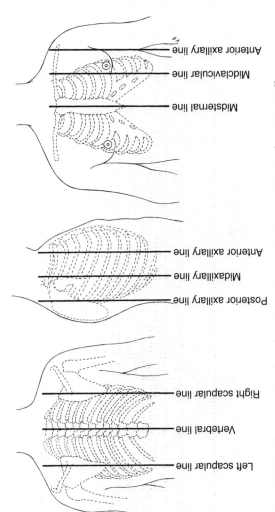

FIGURE 11-3 Chest wall landmarks. (From Potter PA, Perry AG, Stockert PA, Hall A: *Fundamentals of nursing*, ed 8, St. Louis, 2013, Mosby.)

SYSTEMATIC PATTERN FOR PALPATION AND AUSCULTATION

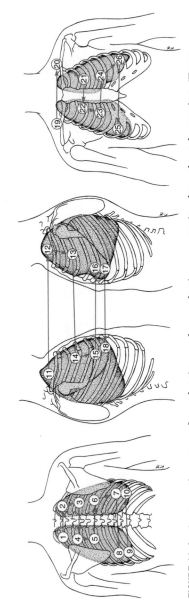

FIGURE 11-4 Systematic pattern for palpation and auscultation—posterior, lateral, and anterior. (From Potter PA, Perry AG, Stockert PA, Hall A: *Fundamentals of nursing,* ed 8, St. Louis, 2013, Mosby.)

NORMAL BREATH SOUNDS

Vesicular Soft, low-pitched sighing over bronchiole and alveoli base on inspiration

Bronchial Moderate, high-pitched sound over trachea

Bronchovesicular Moderate sound over first and second intercostal spaces

Tracheal Loudest and highest pitched of normal breath sounds, harsh and tubular

SIGNS AND SYMPTOMS OF HYPERVENTILATION

- Tachycardia, chest pain, shortness of breath
- Dizziness, lightheadedness, disorientation
- Paresthesia, numbness
- Tinnitus, blurred vision, tetany

SIGNS AND SYMPTOMS OF HYPOVENTILATION

- Dizziness, headache, lethargy
- Disorientation, convulsions, coma
- Decreased ability to follow instructions
- Cardiac arrhythmias, electrolyte imbalance, cardiac arrest

SIGNS AND SYMPTOMS OF HYPOXIA

- Restlessness, anxiety, disorientation
- Decreased concentration, fatigue
- Decreased consciousness, dizziness
- Behavioral changes, pallor
- Increased pulse and blood pressure
- Cardiac arrhythmias, cyanosis, clubbing, dyspnea

Common Abnormalities of the Lung

Type	Characteristics	Assess for
Apnea	Periods of not breathing	Sleep problem, impending death
Bradypnea	<10 breaths/min	Drug overdose, alcohol overdose
Dyspnea	Difficulty breathing	Low hemoglobin, acidosis
Stridor	High-pitched sounds	Obstruction
Tachypnea	>20 breaths/min	Anxiety, fever
Hyperpnea	Increased rate and death	Pain, reaction to altitude
Hyperventilation	Acidosis	Increased rate and depth
Cheyne-Stokes breathing	Alternating periods of hyperpnea and apnea	Impending death
Kussmaul respirations	Extreme rate and depth	Diabetic ketoacidosis, renal failure
Asymmetric	Lungs do not expand equally	Fractured ribs, missing lung, pneumothorax

ABNORMAL AND ADVENTITIOUS SOUNDS

Crackles/rales Fine, crackle-like sounds, usually on inspiration
- **Alveolar** High pitched
- **Bronchial** Low pitched

Rhonchi Coarse, harsh, over fluid (usually on expiration)

Wheezes Squeaky, musical on inspiration or expiration

Friction rub Grating sound of pleurae rubbing together, generally on the anterior side

Assessment Questions Regarding Respiratory Status
Time Pattern
- When did the breathing sound start?
- How long did it last?
- Is there a pattern to the occurrences?

Quality
- How would you describe it?

Relieving factors
- What makes it better?

Aggravating factors
- What makes it worse?

Other
- What other symptoms are also present?
- Is there any coughing?
- Is there any difficulty breathing?

Tests that May Be Ordered for Patients with Abnormal Breath Sounds
- Chest X-ray
- Pulmonary function tests
- Blood tests (including an arterial blood gas)

- CT scan of the chest
- Analysis of a sputum sample

COMMON LUNG DISORDERS
Asthma
Signs and symptoms: Dyspnea, cough, tachypnea
Listen for: Decreased sounds with wheezes

Atelectasis
Signs and symptoms: Tachypnea, cyanosis, use of accessory muscles
Listen for: Decreased sound with crackles

Bronchiectasis
Signs and symptoms: Chronic cough with large amounts of foul-smelling sputum production, coughing up blood, cough worsened by lying on one side, fatigue, shortness of breath worsened by exercise, weight loss, wheezing, paleness, skin discoloration, bluish, breath odor; clubbing of fingers may be present
Listen for: Wheezes and crackles

Bronchitis
Signs and symptoms: Cough with sputum, sore throat and fever, prolonged expiration
Listen for: Prolonged expiration, wheezes, crackles

Cystic Fibrosis (CF)
Signs and symptoms: Recurrent respiratory infections, such as pneumonia or sinusitis; coughing or wheezing; no bowel movements in first 24 to 48 hours of life; and stools that are pale or clay colored, foul-smelling, or that float. Infants may have salty-tasting skin, weight loss, or failure to gain weight normally in childhood; diarrhea; delayed growth; and fatigue.
Listen for: Wheezes and crackles

Emphysema
Signs and symptoms: Dyspnea, cough with sputum
Listen for: Wheezes, rhonchi

Interstitial Lung Disease (ILD)
Signs and symptoms: Shortness of breath during exercise. When the disease is severe and prolonged, heart failure with swelling of the legs may occur.
Listen for: Dry cough without sputum

Neoplasm
Signs and symptoms: Cough with sputum, chest pain
Listen for: Decreased sounds

Pleural Effusion
Signs and symptoms: Pain, dyspnea, pallor, fever, cough
Listen for: Decreased sounds, friction rub

Pneumonia
Signs and symptoms: Chills, productive cough, rapid swallow rate
Listen for: Fine crackles or friction rub

Pneumothorax
Signs and symptoms: Pain, dyspnea, cyanosis, tachypnea
Listen for: Decreased sound on affected side

Pulmonary Edema
Signs and symptoms: Tachypnea, cough, cyanosis, orthopnea, use of accessory muscles
Listen for: Rales, rhonchi, wheezes

Text continued on p. 233

Positions for Postural Drainage

Lung Segment	Position of Patient
Adult	

Bilateral   High Fowler's

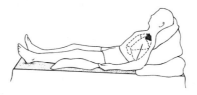

Apical segments
Right upper lobe—
  anterior segment

Supine with head
elevated

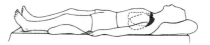

Left upper lobe—
  anterior segment

Supine with head
elevated

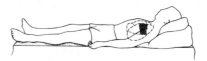

Positions for Postural Drainage—cont'd

Lung Segment	Position of Patient
Right upper lobe— posterior segment	Side lying with right side of chest elevated on pillows

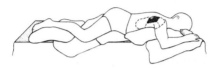

| Left upper lobe— posterior segment | Side lying with left side of chest elevated on pillows |

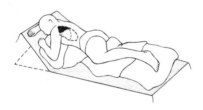

| Right middle lobe— anterior segment | Three-fourths supine position with dependent lung in Trendelenburg position |

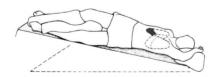

Continued

Positions for Postural Drainage—cont'd

Lung Segment	Position of Patient
Right middle lobe— posterior segment	Prone with thorax and abdomen elevated

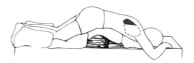

Both lower lobes— anterior segments	Supine in Trendelenburg position

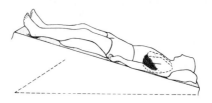

Left lower lobe— lateral segment	Right side lying in Trendelenburg position

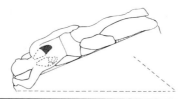

Positions for Postural Drainage—cont'd

Lung Segment	Position of Patient
Right lower lobe— lateral segment	Left side lying in Trendelenburg position

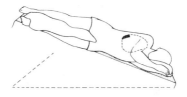

| Right lower lobe— posterior segment | Prone with right side of chest elevated in Trendelenburg position |

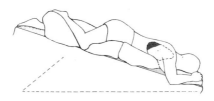

| Both lower lobes— posterior segment | Prone in Trendelenburg position |

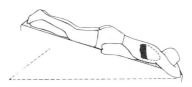

Continued

Positions for Postural Drainage—cont'd

Lung Segment	Position of Patient
Child	
Bilateral—apical segments	Sitting on nurse's lap, leaning slightly forward flexed over pillow

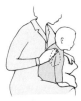

Bilateral—middle anterior segments	Sitting on nurse's lap, leaning against nurse

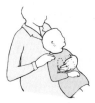

Bilateral lobes—anterior segments	Lying supine on nurse's lap, back supported with pillow

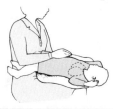

From Potter PA, Perry AG, Stockert PA, Hall A: *Fundamentals of nursing,* ed 8, St. Louis, 2013, Mosby.

OXYGEN THERAPY
Oxygen is a drug so a physician's order is required for use.

Cannula
1 L = 24% oxygen
2 L = 28% oxygen
3 L = 32% oxygen
4 L = 36% oxygen
5 L = 40% oxygen
6 L = 44% oxygen

If patient requires more oxygen than 6 L, a mask may be needed. Humidification may be added for comfort.

Simple Mask
5 to 6 L = 40% oxygen
7 to 8 L = 50% oxygen
10 L = 60% oxygen
Should not be run below 5 L/min.

Partial Rebreathing Mask
6 to 10 L = Up to 80% oxygen

Level of oxygen will depend on patient's overall respiratory and health status. Should not be run below 5 L/min. Reservoir bag should never be fully collapsed.

Non-rebreathing Mask
Will deliver 80% to 100% oxygen. Should not be run below 5 L/min. Reservoir bag should never be fully collapsed.

Pulmonary Functions

Name	Description	Average	Considerations
Tidal volume (VT)	Amount of air inhaled or exhaled	5–10 mL/kg	Decreased in older adults and patients with restrictive lung disease
Residual volume (RV)	Amount of air left in lung after deep exhalation	1200 mL	Increased in patients with chronic obstructive pulmonary disease
Functional residual capacity (PRC)	Air left in lung after normal exhalation	2400 mL	Increased in patients with obstructive lung diseases
Vial capacity (VC)	Amount of air exhaled after maximal inhalation	4800 mL	Decreased with pulmonary edema and atelectasis
Total lung capacity (TLC)	Total air in lungs after maximal inhalation	6000 mL	Decreased with restrictive disease
			Increased with obstructive disease

CHAPTER 12

Endocrine System

For an in-depth study of the endocrine system, consult the following publications:

Lewis SM, et al: *Medical-surgical nursing*, ed 8, St. Louis, 2011, Mosby.

Nugent P, Green J, Hellmer Saul MA, Pelikan P: *Mosby's comprehensive review of nursing for the NCLEX-RN examination*, ed 20, St. Louis, 2012.

Patton K, Thibodeau G: *Structure and function of the human body*, ed 14, St. Louis, 2012, Mosby.

Potter PA, Perry AG, Stockert PA, Hall A: *Fundamentals of nursing,* ed 8, St. Louis, 2013, Mosby.

Weilitz P, Potter PA: *Pocket guide for health assessment*, ed 6, St. Louis, 2007, Mosby.

ENDOCRINE GLANDS AND ASSOCIATED STRUCTURES

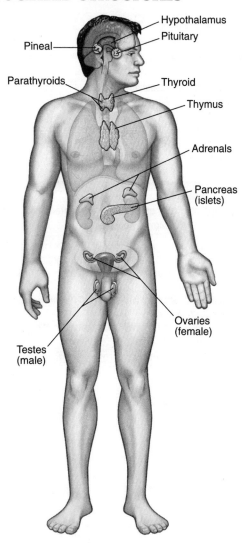

FIGURE 12-1 Endocrine glands. (Modified from Thibodeau G, Patton K: *Structure and function of the human body*, ed 14, St. Louis, 2012, Mosby.)

DIABETES

Types of Diabetes		
	Type 1	**Type 2**
Former Names	Juvenile, insulin dependent diabetes mellitus (IDDM)	Adult-onset, non–insulin dependent diabetes mellitus (NIDDM)
Clinical Information	• 10% to 15% of diabetic cases • Abrupt onset • Autoimmune islet-cell destruction • Generally begins before age 40 years but can occur at any age	• 85% to 90% of diabetic cases • Gradual onset • Insulin resistance or deficiency • Generally begins after age 40 years but can occur earlier
Clinical Manifestations	• Weight loss, increased hunger • Excessive thirst, increased urinary frequency • Possible ketoacidosis • Prone to ketosis • No endogenous insulin	• Fatigue, drowsiness, increased hunger • Blurred vision, increased thirst, urinary frequency • No ketoacidosis • No ketosis • Has endogenous insulin
Management	• Diet very important • Insulin mandatory • Oral hypoglycemic not used	• Diet very important • Insulin needed in 25% of cases • Oral hypoglycemic used in 40% of cases

Blood Glucose Reactions

Insulin Reaction	Diabetic Ketoacidosis
Hypoglycemia (glucose level <60 mg/dL)	Hyperglycemia (glucose level >250 mg/dL)

Causes

• Too much insulin • Skipped or delayed meals • Too much exercise	• Too little insulin • Overeating • Emotional stress illness, infection, surgery, heart attack, stroke, pregnancy

Clinical Manifestations
Early Symptoms

• Sweatiness • Shakiness, weakness • Headache, dizziness • Hunger	• Excessive thirst • Frequent urination • Fatigue • Weakness

Late Symptoms

• Numbness of lips or tongue • Difficulty concentrating • Mood change or irritability • Vision changes, pallor	• Abdominal pain, nausea, vomiting • General aches • Loss of appetite • Flushed, dry skin • Fruity breath, drowsiness

If Not Treated

• Seizures, coma	• Labored breathing, coma

Treatment for Blood Glucose Reactions

Insulin Reaction	**Diabetic Ketoacidosis**
• Hypoglycemia	• Hyperglycemia
• (Glucose level <60 mg/dL)	• (Glucose level >250 mg/dL)

Interventions	

1. Give the patient *one* of the below:
  • 10 to 15 g of sugar or 2 glucose tablets
  • 5 pieces of candy or 4 oz of juice
  • 1 mg IM glucagon
	1. Alert physician.

2. Repeat any *one* of the above in 15 minutes if needed.	2. Monitor blood sugar.
3. Document reaction.	3. Test urine for ketones.
4. Inform physician.	4. Provide IV hydration per physician's orders.
	5. Provide potassium replacements.
	6. Give insulin per physician's order.
	7. Document actions.

INSULIN

Recommendations for Mixing Insulins*

• Mixing insulins requires care and skill to avoid inaccurate dosage and possible contamination. Always be sure to have another nurse double check as you mix the insulins.

---

*Modified from American Diabetes Association: Clinical practice recommendations for insulin administration, *Diabetes Care* 20(suppl 1):46S, 2011.

- When mixing insulin, if one is cloudy, the clear insulin is drawn up first and the cloudy one second.
- If giving any cloudy insulin such as NPH, roll the vial between your hands to mix. DO NOT SHAKE. Shaking will cause air bubbles that will displace insulin and cause inaccurate dosing.
- *Remember:* When mixing insulin, if one is cloudy, it gets drawn up second, but the air is inserted into it first.
- If in doubt, start over. Never allow insulins to mix in the vials. If this happens, discard it and get fresh vials.
- Never administer medications you did not prepare to dispense yourself.
- When mixing short- and long-acting insulins in the same syringe, first draw up the short-acting insulin (regular insulin, which is clear) and then the long-acting insulin (which is cloudy).
- Patients whose blood sugar levels are well controlled on a mixed-insulin dose should maintain their individual routine.
- Insulin should not be mixed with other medications.
- Insulin should not be diluted unless approved by the prescribing physician.
- Rapid-acting insulins that are mixed with NPH or Ultralente insulins should be injected 15 minutes before a meal to promote consistent absorption of insulin.
- Short-acting and Lente insulins should not be mixed unless the patient's blood sugar level is currently under control with this mixture.

Reaction Prevention Tips

Insulin Reaction	**Diabetic Ketoacidosis**
Eat meals at same time each day.	Follow prescribed eating schedule.
If meals are delayed:	Know factors that can raise blood sugar.
• For 1 hr: Drink 4 oz of fruit juice	
• For more than 2 hr: Eat 4 oz of protein	
Take correct insulin as scheduled.	Avoid stress and overwork.
Wear diabetic identification.	Take correct insulin as scheduled.
Check blood sugar as needed.	Wear diabetic identification.
Carry quick-acting sugar at all times.	On sick days:
	• Do not stop insulin.
	• Check urine for ketones every 12 hr.
	• Monitor blood glucose every 2 to 4 hr.
	• Maintain good fluid intake.
	• Alert physician if glucose is >240 mg/dL.

General Patient and Family Information
• With an increase in activity, never omit insulin.
• Before vacations, call physician to see whether insulin dose needs adjusting.
• Know insulin peaks and how body reacts to insulin highs and lows.
• Inform family and friends of possible reactions and how to treat them.

	Types of Insulin					
Type	Name	Color	Onset	Peak		Duration (hr)
Rapid-acting	Humalog (Insulin Lispro)	Clear	5–10 min	30–90 min		3–5
	Novolog (Insulin Aspart)	Clear	5–10 min	40–50 min		3–5
Short-acting	Humulin-R (insulin regular)	Clear	30 min	1–2 hr		4–6
Intermediate-acting	Humulin-N (insulin NPH)	Cloudy	1–2 hr	4–6 hr		8–24
	Novolin-L (insulin Lente)	Cloudy	1–3 hr	6–15 hr		10–24
Long acting	Humulin-U (insulin Ultralente)	Cloudy	4–6 hr	8–30 hr		24–36
	Lantus (insulin glargine)	Clear	Within a few minutes	Adsorbed into the blood slowly, so there is no time of greatest effect		24

Insulin Pens

Most insulin pens fall into one of two groups: reusable pens and disposable pens.

- A **reusable insulin pen** must be loaded with a cartridge. When the cartridge is empty, it is thrown it away, and a new cartridge is loaded. A reusable pen can often be used for several years.
- **Disposable insulin pens** come filled with insulin and are thrown away when empty. Disposable pens are generally more convenient than reusable pens, but they usually cost more to use than reusable pens and cartridges.

Advantages

- Insulin pens are portable, discreet, and convenient for injections away from home.
- They save time because there is no need to draw up insulin from a bottle.
- They let you set an accurate dose by the turn of a dosage dial, which may make it easier for people who have vision or dexterity problems.

Disadvantages

- Insulin in pens and cartridges is often more expensive than insulin in bottles.
- One to two units of insulin is often lost when the pen is primed before each injection.
- Not all insulin types are available for use in insulin pen cartridges.
- Insulin pens do not let you mix insulin types.
- Insulin pens should only be used for self-injection. There is no way to completely protect the person giving the injection from getting accidentally stuck by the needle.

Factors to Consider when Choosing a Pen
- Insurance: Will the patient's insurance pay for the type of pen needed?
- The number of units of insulin that the pen holds when full.
- The largest size dose that can be injected with the pen.
- The size of the numbers on the pen dose dial and whether they are magnified.
- The amount of strength and dexterity required to operate the pen.
- How to correct a mistake if you dial the wrong dose into the pen.

Classes of Oral Hypoglycemic Agents		
Class Agent	**Peak**	**Duration**
Sulfonylureas First Generation		
Acetohexamide (Dymelor)	1.3–8 hr	12–24 hr
Chlorpropamide (Diabinese)	1 hr	24–60 hr
Tolbutamide (Orinase)	5–8 hr	6–12 hr
Tolazamide (Tolinase)	4–6 hr	12–24 hr
Second Generation		
Glipizide (Glucotrol)	1–3 hr	10–24 hr
Glyburide (DiaBeta, Micronase, Glynase)	2–8 hr	24 hr
Glimepiride (Amaryl)	2–3 hr	24 hr
Biguanides		
Metformin (Glucophage) [Biguanides]	1–3 hr	9–17 hr

Classes of Oral Hypoglycemic Agents—cont'd		
Class Agent	**Peak**	**Duration**
Alpha Inhibitors		
Acarbose (Precose)	1 hr	14–24 hr
Miglitol (Glyset)	2–3 hr	24 hr
Thiazolidinediones		
Pioglitazone (Actos)	2 hr	16–24
Meglitinides		
Nateglinide (Starlix) [Meglitinides]	0–1 hr	2–3 hr
Repaglinide (Prandin) [Meglitinides]	60–90 min	<4 hr

ADRENAL GLANDS

Cushing syndrome	Addison disease
Hyperfunction	Hypofunction
Clinical Manifestations	
Excessive cortisol production	Inadequate cortisol production
Increased adrenocorticotropic hormone (ACTH) from pituitary	Insufficient ACTH from pituitary
Increased protein catabolism	Flaccid muscles or paralysis
Muscle wasting and fragile skin	Muscle weakness and anorexia
Osteoporosis and compression fractures	Nausea or vomiting and diarrhea
Bruises easily or poor healing	Abdominal pain
Obesity, moon face, buffalo hump	Weight loss
Hyperglycemia and worsening of diabetes	Frequent hypoglycemia

Decreased immunity	Decreased cardiac output
Sodium and water retention	Hyponatremia and hypo-osmolality
Edema or hypertension	Hypotension and arrhythmias
Hypokalemia or hypochloremia	Hyperkalemia
Renal calculi hypercalcemia	Hypercalcemia
Irritability	Lethargy
Anxiety	Depression

PITUITARY GLAND*

Hyperpituitarism

Clinical information. This disorder is generally caused by tumors, which lead to an increase in hormone levels. The most common hormones involved are the following:

- **GH** Growth hormone, which causes gigantism
- **ACTH** Adrenocorticotropic hormone (corticotropin), which causes Cushing disease
- **TSH** Thyroid-stimulating hormone, which causes hyperthyroidism
- **LH** Luteinizing hormone
- **FSH** Follicle-stimulating hormone

Hypopituitarism

Clinical information. This disorder is usually caused by tumors, necrosis, or glandular dysfunction, leading to a decrease in hormone levels. The most common problems associated with hypopituitarism are:

- **Dwarfism** Caused by a decreased GH
- **Hypophysectomy** The removal or destruction of the pituitary gland

---

*Specific problems, signs, and symptoms will depend on the hormone involved.

- **Postpartum necrosis** Caused by hypotension after delivery
- **Functional disorders** Caused by starvation or anemia

THYROID GLAND

Hyperthyroidism	Hypothyroidism
Clinical Manifestations	
Increased body metabolism	Decreased body metabolism
Nervousness or restlessness	Lethargy and headaches
Short attention span	Memory deficit
Tachycardia (>100 beats/min; bounding heard sounds)	Bradycardia (<60 beats/min; weak heart sounds)
Increased blood pressure	Decreased blood pressure
Reduced vital capacity	Lowered respiratory rate
Skin warm, moist, and smooth	Skin cool, dry, and rough
Hair fine, nails soft	Coarse hair, brittle nails
Weakness and fatigue	Weakness and fatigue
Demineralization of bones	Stiff joints
Hypercalcemia	Mild proteinuria
Brisk reflexes	Decreased reflexes
Increased appetite or weight loss	Decreased appetite or weight gain
Muscle wasting	Muscular stiffness
Diabetes worsens	Diabetic patients need less insulin
Increased stools	Constipation
Increased libido	Decreased libido
Decreased fertility	Decreased fertility
Higher body temperature	Lower body temperature

Digestive System

For in-depth study of the digestive system, consult the following publications:

Lewis SM, et al: *Medical-surgical nursing*, ed 8, St. Louis, 2011, Mosby.

Nugent P, Green J, Hellmer Saul MA, Pelikan P: *Mosby's comprehensive review of nursing for the NCLEX-RN examination*, ed 20, St. Louis, 2012, Mosby.

Patton K, Thibodeau G: *Structure and function of the human body*, ed 14, St. Louis, 2012, Mosby.

Potter PA, Perry AG, Stockert PA, Hall A: *Fundamentals of nursing,* ed 8, St. Louis, 2013, Mosby

Weilitz P, Potter PA: *Pocket guide for health assessment*, ed 6, St. Louis, 2007, Mosby

DIGESTIVE SYSTEM AND ASSOCIATED STRUCTURES

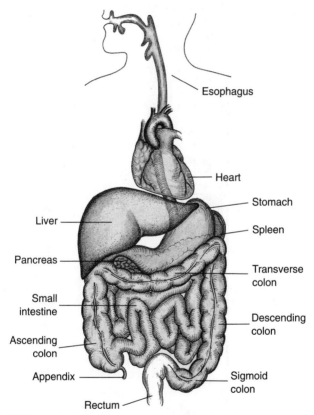

FIGURE 13-1 Digestive system and associated structures. (From Potter PA, Perry AG, Stockert PA, Hall A: *Fundamentals of nursing,* ed 8, St. Louis, 2013, Mosby.)

Types of Diets

Type	Description	Patient Complaint
Regular	Has all essentials; no restrictions	No special diet needed
Clear liquid	Broth, tea, clear soda, strained juices, gelatin	Recovery from surgery or very ill
Full liquid	Clear liquids plus milk products, eggs	Transition from clear to regular diet
Soft	Soft consistency and mild spice	Difficulty swallowing
Mechanical soft	Regular diet but chopped or ground	Difficulty chewing
Bland	No spicy food	Ulcers or colitis
Low residue	No bulky food, apples, or nuts	Rectal disease
High calorie	High protein, vitamin, and fat	Malnourished

Low calorie	Decreased fat, no whole milk, cream eggs, complex carbohydrates	Obese
Diabetic	Balance of protein, carbohydrates, fat	Insulin–food imbalance
High protein	Meat, fish, milk, cheese, poultry, eggs	Tissue repair, underweight
Low fat	Little butter, cream, whole milk, or eggs	Gallbladder, liver, or heart disease
Low cholesterol	Little meat or cheese	Need to decrease fat intake
Low sodium	No salt added during cooking	Heart or renal disease
Salt free	No salt	Heart or renal disease
Tube feeding	Formulas or liquid food	Oral surgery, oral or esophageal cancers, inability to eat or swallow

Types of Nutrients		
Type	**Function**	**Food Sources**
Carbohydrate	Energy, body temperature	*Simple:* sugars, fruits, nuts *Complex:* grains, potatoes milk
Protein	Tissue growth, tissue repair	Meat, fish, eggs, milk, poultry, beans, peas, nuts
Fat	Energy and repair, carries vitamins A and D	Animal fat, meat, nuts, milk, fish, poultry
Water	Carries nutrients, regulates body processes, lubricates joints	Liquids, most fruits and vegetables

Minerals		
Type	**Function**	**Food Sources**
Calcium	Renews bones and teeth, regulates heart and nerves	Milk, green vegetables, cheese, salmon, legumes
Phosphorus	Renews bones and teeth, maintains nerve function	Cheese, oats, meat, milk, fish, poultry, nuts
Iron	Renews hemoglobin	Meat, eggs, liver, flour, yellow or green vegetables
Iodine	Regulates thyroid	Table salt, seafood
Magnesium	Component of enzymes	Grains, green vegetables
Sodium	Maintains water balance, nerve function	Salt, cured meats
Potassium	Maintains nerve function	Meat, milk, vegetables
Chloride	Formation of gastric juices	Salt
Zinc	Component of enzymes	Meat, seafood

Vitamins

Type	Function	Food Sources
A (retinol)	Helps eyes, skin, hair; fights infection	Yellow fruits and vegetables, liver, kidneys, fish
B₁ (thiamine)	Maintains nerves, aids carbohydrate function	Bread, cereal, beans, peas, pork, liver, eggs, milk
B₂ (riboflavin)	Maintains skin, mouth, nerve functions	Milk, cheese, eggs, cereal, dark green vegetables
B₃ (niacin)	Oxidation of proteins and carbohydrates	Meat, fish, poultry, eggs, nuts, bread, cereal
B₁₂	Aids muscles, nerves, heart, metabolism	Organ meats, milk
C (ascorbic acid)	Maintains integrity of cells, repairs tissue	Citrus fruits, tomatoes, green vegetables, potatoes
D	Enables body to use calcium and phosphorus	Milk, margarine, fish, liver, eggs
F	Antioxidant	Peanuts, vegetable oils
K	Aids in blood clotting	Green leafy vegetables

Caloric Increase Needed For Select Injury Factors	
Injury	**% Caloric Increase**
Minor surgery	10
Mild infection	20
Moderate infection	40
Severe infection	60
Congestive heart failure	30
Cancer therapy	30
Pulmonary disease	30
Wound healing	20–60
Long bone fracture	30–50

TWO TYPES OF MALNUTRITION*
Marasmus
Caused by decreased caloric intake
- Takes months to years to develop
- Individuals appear thin and malnourished
- Weight loss present
- Serum albumin and transferrin levels normal
- Mortality rate low unless from underlying disease

Kwashiorkor*
Caused by decreased protein intake or stress
- Can be caused by trauma or infection
- Takes only weeks to develop
- Individuals appear normal and well nourished

---

*Modified from Kobriger Presents. Available at http://www.kobriger.com.

- Weight loss may be minimal or masked by edema
- Serum albumin and transferrin levels are decreased
- Mortality rate high because of decreased wound healing
- High risk of infection

Comparing Peptic Ulcers	
Gastric Ulcers	**Duodenal Ulcers**
Located in the antrum of stomach	Located in the first 1 to 2 cm of the duodenum
Generally occurs in people ages 45 to 70 years	Generally occurs in people ages 40 to 60 years
Most common ulcer in people older than 65 years old	Most common ulcer in people younger than 65 years old
More common in women	More common in men
Higher mortality rate than duodenal ulcers	Lower mortality rate than gastric ulcers
Less common than duodenal ulcers	Four times more prevalent than gastric ulcers
Risk factors are stress, drugs, alcohol, smoking, and gastritis	Risk factors are chronic obstructive pulmonary disease, alcohol, cirrhosis, pancreatitis, smoking, renal failure, stress

Comparing Peptic Ulcers—cont'd	
Gastric Ulcers	**Duodenal Ulcers**
Pain occurs 1 to 2 hours after eating	Pain occurs after eating and at night
Pain felt high in epigastrium	Pain in midepigastric area
Pain may be described as heartburn	Pain is described in the back
Pain relieved by food or liquids	Pain relieved by milk or antacids
May cause weight loss	May cause weight gain
High recurrence rate	Recurs seasonally (spring and fall)
Risk of malignancy	Rarely malignant
High risk of hemorrhage	High risk of perforation

ALTERED BOWEL ELIMINATION PATTERNS
Constipation
Presence of large quantity of dry, hard feces that is difficult to expel; frequency of bowel movements is not a factor.

Causes Reabsorption of too much water in the lower bowel as a result of medication such as narcotics, ignoring the urge to defecate, immobility, chronic laxative abuse, low fluid intake, low fiber intake, aging, postoperative conditions, or pregnancy

Remedies Increase fluids, fiber cereals, fruits and vegetables, exercise, and avoid cheese.

Impaction
Hard, dry stool embedded in rectal folds; may have liquid stool passing around impaction.
Causes Poor bowel habits, immobility, inadequate food or fluids, or barium in rectum
Remedies Digitally remove impaction, increase fluids and fiber, increase exercise, and institute bowel program.

Diarrhea
Expulsion of fecal matter that contains too much water.
Causes Infection, anxiety, stress, medications, too many laxatives at one time, or food or drug allergies or reactions
Remedies Add bulk or fiber to diet, maintain fluids and electrolytes, eat smaller amounts of food at one time, add cheese or bananas to diet, and rest after eating.

Incontinence
Inability to hold feces in rectum because of impairment of sphincter control.
Causes Surgery, cancer, radiation treatment of rectum, paralysis, or aging
Remedies Bowel training, regular meal times, regular elimination patterns

Abdominal Distention

Tympanites, or enlargement of the abdomen with gas or air as a result of excessive swallowing of air, eating gas-producing foods, or an inability to expel gas.

Causes Constipation, fecal impaction, or postoperative conditions

Remedies Rectal tube can be used to expel air; increase ambulation, and change position in bed.

Obstruction

Occurs when the lumen of the bowel narrows or closes completely.

Causes External compression can be caused by tumor; internal narrowing can be caused by impacted feces.

Remedies Remove impaction or tumor.

Ileus (Paralytic Ileus)

Occurs when the bowel has decreased motility.

Causes Surgery, long-term narcotic use, or complete obstruction

Remedies. Medical intervention for physical obstructions. Specific action depend on the cause of the ileus.

	Fecal Characteristics		
Characteristic	Normal	Abnormal	Assess for
Color	Brown	Clay or white	Bile obstruction
		Black or tarry	Upper GI bleeding, iron
		Red	Lower GI bleeding, beets
		Pale	Malabsorption of fat
		Green	Infection
Consistency	Moist	Hard	Constipation, dehydration
	Formed	Loose	Diet, diarrhea, medications
		Watery	Infection
		Liquid	Impaction
Odor	Aromatic	Pungent	Infection, blood
Frequency	1–2 times per day	5 times per day	Infection, diet
	Once every 3 days	Once every 6 days	Constipation, activity, medications
Shape	Cylindric	Narrow, "ribbon-like"	Obstruction

GI, gastrointestinal.

FOODS AND THEIR EFFECT ON FECAL OUTPUT

To thicken stool, a person should eat:
- Bananas, rice, bread, potatoes
- Creamy peanut butter, applesauce
- Cheese, yogurt, pasta, pretzels
- Tapioca, marshmallows

To loosen stool, a person should eat:
- Chocolate, raw fruits and vegetables
- Spiced foods, greasy or fried foods
- Prunes, grapes, leafy green vegetables

To decrease gas, a person should avoid:
- Beans, beer, sodas
- Cucumbers, cabbage, onions, spinach
- Brussels sprouts, broccoli, cauliflower
- Most dairy products, corn, radishes

TYPES OF CATHARTICS

Bulk forming Increases fluids and bulk in the intestines, which stimulates peristalsis. An increase in fluid is needed
Example: Metamucil

Emollient Softens and delays drying of stool
Example: Liquid petrolatum

Irritant Stimulates peristalsis by irritating bowel mucosa and decreasing water absorption
Example: Castor oil

Moistening (stool softeners) Increase water in the bowel
Example: Colace

Saline When salt is in the bowel, the water will remain in the bowel as well. (Avoid use in patients with impaired renal function.)
Example: Milk of magnesia (MOM), Epsom salts

Suppository Stimulates bowel and softens stool

ANTIDIARRHEAL MEDICATIONS
Absorbent Absorbs gas
Astringent Shrinks inflamed tissues
Demulcent Coats and protects bowel

TYPES OF ENEMAS
Carminative Used to expel flatus
Cleansing Stimulates peristalsis; irritates bowel by distention. (Use 1 L of fluid; have patient hold it as long as possible.)
Colonic irrigation Used to expel flatus
Hypertonic Phosphates irritate bowel and draw fluid into bowel through osmosis (90–120 mL; hold for 10–15 min)
Hypotonic Tap water (1 L; hold for 15 min); avoid with cardiac patients
Medicated Contains a therapeutic agent (e.g., Kayexalate to treat high potassium levels)
Retention Oil given to soften stool (hold for 1 hr)
Saline Draws fluid into the bowel (9 mL of sodium to 1 L of water; hold for 15 min).
Soapsuds Irritates and distends bowel (5 mL of soap to 1 L of water; hold for 15 min); use only Castile soaps

COMMON TYPES OF OSTOMIES*
Ileostomy
Effluent A continuous discharge that is soft and wet. The output is somewhat odorous and contains intestinal enzymes that are irritating to peristomal skin.
Skin barrier option Highly desirable for peristomal skin protection
Pouch option. Pouch necessary at all times

Type of pouch. Drainable or closed-end for specific needs
Need for irrigation None

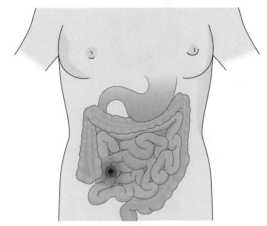

(From Perry AG, Potter PA, Elkin MK: *Nursing interventions & clinical skills*, ed 5, St. Louis, 2012, Mosby.)

Transverse Colostomy
Effluent Usually semiliquid or very soft. Occasionally, transverse colostomy discharge is firm. Output is usually malodorous and can irritate peristomal skin. Double-barreled colostomies have two openings. Loop colostomies have one opening but two tracks—the active (proximal), which discharges fecal matter, and the inactive (distal), which discharges mucus.
Skin barrier option. Highly desirable for peristomal skin protection
Pouch option Pouch necessary at all times
Type of pouch Drainable or closed end for specific needs
Need for irrigation None

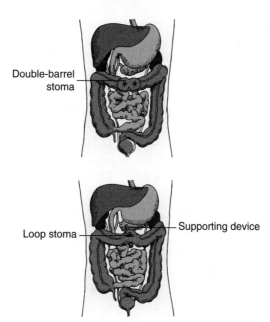

Double-barrel stoma

Loop stoma

Supporting device

(From Potter PA, Perry AG, Stockert PA, Hall A: *Fundamentals of nursing*, ed 8, St. Louis, 2013, Mosby.)

Descending Colostomy or Sigmoid Colostomy

Effluent Semisolid from descending colostomy. Firm from sigmoid colostomy. On discharge, there is an odor. Discharge is irritating if left in contact with skin around stoma. Frequency of output is unpredictable and varies with each person.

Skin barrier option May be used for peristomal skin protection if pouch is worn

Pouch option Pouch should be worn if person does not irrigate

Type of pouch Drainable, closed end, or stoma cap

Need for irrigation Yes, as instructed by enterostomal (ET) nurse or physician

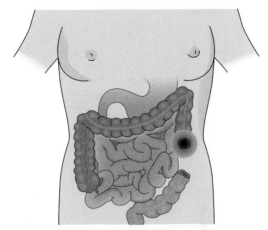

(From Perry AG, Potter PA, Elkin MK: *Nursing interventions & clinical skills*, ed 5, St. Louis, 2012, Mosby.)

Urinary Diversion (Ileal Loop, Ileal, or Colonic Conduit)

Effluent Urine only. Output is constant. Mucus is expelled with urine. Mild odor unless there is a urinary tract infection. Urine is irritating when in contact with skin. Segment of ileum or colon is used to construct stoma.

Skin barrier option Highly desirable for peristomal skin protection

Pouch option Pouch necessary at all times

Type of pouch Drainable pouch with spout

Need for irrigation None

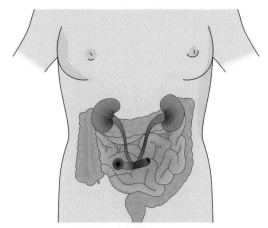

(From Perry AG, Potter PA, Elkin MK: *Nursing interventions & clinical skills*, ed 5, St. Louis, 2012, Mosby.)

Continent Ileostomy

Effluent Fluid bowel secretions are collected in a reservoir surgically constructed out of the lower part of the small intestine. Gas and feces are emptied via a surgically created leak-free nipple valve through which a catheter is inserted into the reservoir. For maximum efficiency and comfort, the reservoir is usually emptied four or five times daily. Daily schedule for catheterization should be recommended by the ET nurse or physician.

Skin barrier option None; an absorbent pad provides peristomal skin protection

Pouch option None, but catheter should be available at all times.

Type of pouch None; a drainable pouch can be applied if there is leakage of stool between intubations

Need for irrigation Occasionally to liquefy thick fecal matter, the pouch can be irrigated with 1 to 1.5 oz of saline or water. Specific care should be clarified by the ET nurse or physician.

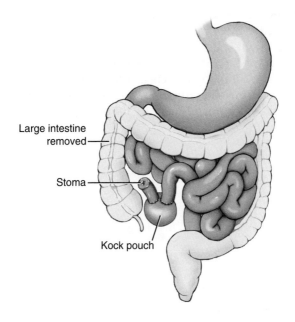

Large intestine removed

Stoma

Kock pouch

Continent Urostomy
Effluent Urine is maintained in a surgically constructed ileal pouch until emptied by means of a catheter inserted into the stoma. Uses two nipple valves—one to prevent the reflux of urine from backing up into the kidneys and the other to keep urine in the pouch until eliminated. Pouch is drained approximately four times daily. Daily schedule for pouch catheterization should be recommended by the ET nurse or physician.
Skin barrier option None; an absorbent pad provides peristomal skin protection
Pouch option None, but a catheter should be available at all times

Type of pouch None; a urostomy pouch can be applied if there is leakage of urine between intubations

Need for irrigation Irrigate daily with 1 to 1.5 oz of saline solution and repeat several times as needed until the returns are clear. Specific care should be clarified by the ET nurse or physician.

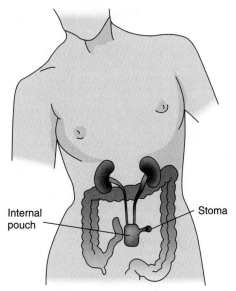

Internal pouch · Stoma

(From Perry AG, Potter PA: *Clinical nursing skills & techniques*, ed 7, St. Louis, 2010, Mosby.)

CHAPTER 14

Urinary System

For an in-depth study of the urinary system,
consult the following publications:

Lewis SM, et al: *Medical-surgical nursing*, ed 8, St. Louis, 2011, Mosby.

Nugent P, Green J, Hellmer Saul MA, Pelikan P: *Mosby's comprehensive review of nursing for the NCLEX-RN examination*, ed 20, St. Louis, 2012, Mosby.

Patton K, Thibodeau G: *Structure and function of the human body*, ed 14, St. Louis, 2012, Mosby.

Potter PA, Perry AG, Stockert PA, Hall A: *Fundamentals of nursing,* ed 8, St. Louis, 2013, Mosby.

Weilitz P, Potter PA: *Pocket guide for health assessment*, ed 6, St. Louis, 2007, Mosby.

ORGANS OF THE URINARY SYSTEM

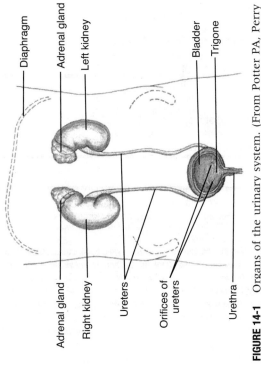

FIGURE 14-1 Organs of the urinary system. (From Potter PA, Perry AG, Stockert PA, Hall A: *Fundamentals of nursing,* ed 8, St. Louis, 2013, Mosby.)

Altered Urinary Patterns

Pattern	Description	Assess for
Anuria	No urination	Renal failure, dehydration, obstruction
Dysuria	Painful urination	Infection, injury, frequency, blood
Frequency	Voiding small amounts	Infection, injury, pregnancy, stress, intake
Incontinence	Difficulty with control	Infection, injury, distended bladder
Nocturia	Urinating at night	Infection, injury, pregnancy, stress, intake
Oliguria	Little urination	Infection, injury, elevated BUN, dehydration, kidney, disease
Polyuria	Increased urination	Infection, injury, alcohol, diabetes, caffeine, diuretics, increased thirst, dehydration
Retention	Holding on to urine	Infection, injury, pain, distended bladder, medications, restlessness, surgical, complications
Residual	No urination Urine remaining in bladder after voiding	Infection, distention, pain, injury
Urgency	Urgent and immediate need to void	Infection

BUN, Blood urea nitrogen.

	Urinary Incontinence		
Type	**Description**	**Causes**	**Symptoms**
Function	Involuntary and unpredictable with intact urinary and nervous systems	Changes in environment or cognitive deficits	Urge to void that causes loss of urine
Reflex	Involuntary and occurring at predictable intervals	Anesthesia, medications, spinal cord dysfunction	Lack of urge to void
Stress	Intraabdominal pressure causes leakage	Coughing, laughing, obesity, pregnancy, weak muscles	Urgency and frequency
Urge	Involuntary passage of urine with strong urgency	Small bladder capacity, bladder irritation, alcohol, caffeine	Bladder spasms, urgency and frequency
Total	Uncontrolled and continuous loss of urine	Neuropathy, trauma, fistula between bladder and vagina	Constant flow, nocturia, unaware of incontinence

	Urine Characteristics		
Characteristics	**Normal**	**Abnormal**	**Asses for**
Amount in 24 hr	1200 mL	<1200 mL	Renal failure
	1500 mL	>1500 mL	Fluid intake
Color	Straw	Amber	Dehydration, fluid intake
		Light straw	Overhydration
		Orange	Medications
		Red	Blood, injury, medications
Consistency	Clear	Cloudy, thick	Infection
Odor	Faint	Offensive	Infection, medications
Sterile	Yes	Organisms	Infection, poor hygiene
pH	4.5	<4.5	Infection
	8.0	>8.0	Diabetes, starvation, dehydration
Specific gravity	1.010	<1.010	Diabetes insipidus, kidney failure
	1.025	>1.025	Diabetes, underhydration
Glucose	None	Present	Diabetes
Ketones	None	Present	Diabetes, starvation, vomiting
Blood	None	Present	Tumors, injury, kidney disease

MEDICATIONS THAT MAY DISCOLOR URINE

Dark Yellow
- Vitamin B_2

Orange
- Sulfonamide
- Phenazopyridine HCl (Pyridium)
- Warfarin (Coumadin)

Pink or Red
- Thorazine
- Ex-Lax
- Phenytoin (Dilantin)

Green or Blue
- Amitriptyline
- Methylene blue
- Triamterene (Dyrenium)

Brown or Black
- Iron
- Levodopa
- Nitrofurantoin
- Metronidazole (Flagyl)

REASONS FOR URINARY CATHETERS

Intermittent
- Relieve bladder distention
- Obtain a sterile specimen
- Assessment of residual urine
- Long-term management of patients with spinal cord injuries and disorders

Short-Term Indwelling
- After surgery
- Prevention of urethral obstruction
- Measurement of output in bedridden patients
- Bladder irrigation

Long-Term Indwelling
- Severe urinary retention
- Avoidance of skin rashes or infections

Types And Sizes of Urinary Catheters	
Type	**Size**
Single lumen	8–18 Fr*
Double lumen	
With inflated balloon	8–10 Fr with 3-mL balloon
	12–30 Fr with 5- to 30-mL balloon
Common male sizes	16–18 Fr
Common female sizes	12–16 Fr

Triple lumen is used for continuous bladder irrigation. Coudé-tip catheter is used for men with an enlarged prostate gland.
*Fr, French.

PREVENTING URINARY CATHETER INFECTIONS

- Use good handwashing techniques before handling.
- Avoid raising the drainage bag above the bladder.
- Allow urine to drain freely into the bag.
- Perform good perineal care on the patient.
- Secure the catheter per procedure.
- Empty the drainage bag at least every 8 hours.
- Avoid kinking the tubing.
- Clean the spigot thoroughly before and after use.
- Avoid dragging the drainage bag on the floor.

TIMED URINE TESTS

Quantitative albumin (24 hr) Determines albumin lost in urine as a result of kidney disease, hypertension, or heart failure

Amino acid (24 hr) Determines the presence of congenital kidney disease

Amylase (2, 12, and 24 hr) Determines the presence of disease of the pancreas

Chloride (24 hr) Determines loss of chloride in cardiac patients on low-salt or no-salt diets

Concentration and dilution Determines the presence of diseases of the kidney tubules

Creatinine clearance (12 and 24 hr) Determines the ability of the kidneys to clear creatinine

Estriol (24 hr) Measures this hormone in women with high-risk pregnancies because of diabetes

Glucose tolerance (12 and 24 hr) Determines malfunctions of the liver and pancreas

17-Hydroxycorticosteroid (24 hr) Determines functioning ability of the adrenal cortex

Urinalysis (random times) Determines levels of bacteria, white blood cell count, red blood cell count, pH, specific gravity, protein, and bilirubin

Urine culture (random times) Determines the amount and type of bacteria in the urine

Urine sensitivity (random times) Determines the antibiotics to which the microorganisms will be sensitive or resistant

Urobilinogen (random times) Determines the presence of obstruction of the biliary tract

CHAPTER 15

Reproductive System

Assessing Sexual History (p. 278)
Medications That Affect Sexual Performance (p. 279)

For an in-depth study of the urinary system,
consult the following publications:

Lewis SM, et al: *Medical-surgical nursing*, ed 8, St. Louis, 2011, Mosby.
Nugent P, Green J, Hellmer Saul MA, Pelikan P: *Mosby's comprehensive review of nursing for the NCLEX-RN examination*, ed 20, St. Louis, 2012, Mosby.
Patton K, Thibodeau G: *Structure and function of the human body*, ed 14, St. Louis, 2012, Mosby.
Potter PA, Perry AG, Stockert PA, Hall A: *Fundamentals of nursing,* ed 8, St. Louis, 2013, Mosby.
Weilitz P, Potter PA: *Pocket guide to health assessment*, ed 6, St. Louis, 2007, Mosby.

ASSESSING SEXUAL HISTORY
Include the following information:

Male
Practice of testicular examinations
Last prostate examination and results
Knowledge of deficit
Concerns or difficulty with sexual activities
Body image concerns
Concerns regarding the effect of treatment on
    future sexual activities
Attitudes regarding sex

Female
Last menstrual cycle
Onset of menopause
Knowledge deficit
Number of pregnancies, children, and miscarriages
Body image concerns
Practice of breast self-examination
Last mammogram and results
Last Pap smear and pelvic examination and
    results
Any concerns or difficulty with sexual activities
Concerns regarding the effect of treatment on
    future sexual activities
Attitudes regarding sex

MEDICATIONS THAT AFFECT SEXUAL PERFORMANCE*

Neurologic Drugs

Anticonvulsants Lethargy, weight changes, menstrual changes

Antidepressants Blurred vision, confusion, loss of libido, failure to reach orgasm, and erectile problems

Hallucinogens Muscle spasms, loss of coordination, aggressive behavior, catatonic syndrome

Tranquilizers Drowsiness, confusion, and decreased desire

Cardiac Drugs

Antiarrhythmic Dizziness, headaches, weakness, fatigue, sexual dysfunction

Antianginal Headache, lightheadedness, nausea, vomiting, or weakness

Antihypertensives Loss of libido, weakness

Diuretics Dizziness, headaches, weakness

Endocrine Drugs

Corticosteroids Mood changes, menstrual changes, headaches, weakness

Hypoglycemics Dizziness, drowsiness, heartburn, nausea, constipation, frequent urination

Gastrointestinal Drugs

Cimetidine Impotence, dizziness, nausea

Ranitidine Impotence, decrease libido

---

*Consult a drug reference book for more information on specific drugs and their side effects.

Common Male Reproductive Disorders

Disorder	Description	Assess for
Hydrocele	Collection of fluid in testes	Pain, swelling
Spermatocele	Cystic mass of the epididymis	Pain, swelling
Varicocele	Dilation of spermatic vein	Pain, swelling
Torsion of spermatic cord	Kinking of cord	Sexual dysfunction
Cancer	Testicular cancer	Enlarged testes, lump
	Penile cancer	Growths, fatigue, weight loss, dysfunction
	Prostate cancer	Urinary dysfunction
Urethritis	Inflammation of urethra	Urgency, frequency, burning with urination
Prostatitis	Inflammation of prostate	Pain, fever, dysuria, urethral drainage
Epididymitis	Inflammation of epididymis	Scrotal pain, edema
Benign prostatic hypertrophy	Enlarged prostate	Dysuria, pain

Common Female Reproductive Disorders		
Disorder	**Description**	**Assess for**
Uterine prolapse	Displacement of uterus	Dysmenorrhea, backache, pelvic pain
Cystocele	Bladder herniation into vagina	Backache, stress, incontinence
Rectocele	Rectum herniation into vagina	Constipation, hemorrhoids
Ovarian cyst	Enlarged ovaries	Menstrual changes, abdominal swelling
Endometriosis	Seeding of endometrial cells into pelvis	Pain, infertility, menstrual changes
Cervical polyps	Benign tumor	Bleeding between periods and with intercourse, increased cervical mucosa
Cancer	Cervical cancer	Spotting, pain
	Uterine cancer	Pain, abdominal fullness, postmenopausal bleeding
	Ovarian cancer	Ascites, fatigue, weight loss, abdominal fullness

	Sexually Transmitted Infections*		
Organism	Infections	Symptoms	Treatment
Bacteria	Gonorrhea, chancroid, granuloma	Purulent discharge	Penicillin
Spirochete	Syphilis	Stage 1: chancre	Penicillin
		Stage 2: body rash	
		Stage 3: tumors, nerve damage, cardiac damage	
Chlamydia	Nongonococcal urethritis, cervicitis, epididymitis, pelvic inflammatory disease	Purulent drainage, fever, chills, pain, and vomiting	Antibiotics
Virus	Herpes, CMV (HPV)	Vesicles	Acyclovir
	AIDS	Pulmonary infections	Antibiotics, supportive care
Protozoa	Trichomoniasis	Itching, greenish discharge	Vinegar
Yeast	Candidiasis	Itching, white, cheesy discharge	Nystatin, miconazole

*Sexually transmitted infections are any disorders that can be transmitted from one person to another through sexual contact.

CMV, cytomegalovirus; HPV, human papillomavirus.

CHAPTER 16

Tests and Procedures

Arterial Blood Gases (p. 288)
Electrolyte Imbalances (p. 289)
Fluid Volume Imbalances (p. 291)
Diagnostic Tests (p. 295)

For an in-depth study of tests and procedures,
consult the following publications:

Lewis SM, et al: *Medical-surgical nursing*, ed 8, St. Louis, 2011, Mosby.

Nugent P, Green J, Hellmer Saul MA, Pelikan P: *Mosby's comprehensive review of nursing for the NCLEX-RN examination*, ed 20, St. Louis, 2012, Mosby.

Myers JL: *Quick medication administration reference*, ed 3, St. Louis, 1998, Mosby.

Pagana KD, Pagana TJ: *Mosby's diagnostic and laboratory test reference*, ed 10, St. Louis, 2010, Mosby.

Patton K, Thibodeau G: *Structure and function of the human body*, ed 14, St. Louis, 2012, Mosby.

Potter PA, Perry AG, Stockert PA, Hall A: *Fundamentals of nursing,* ed 8, St. Louis, 2013, Mosby.

Weilitz P, Potter PA: *Pocket guide for health assessment*, ed 6, St. Louis, 2007, Mosby.

Laboratory Values*	
Laboratory Test	**Reference Range**

Complete Blood Cell Count

Red blood cells (RBCs)	Males: 4.25–6.1 × 10 mL
	Females: 3.6–5.4 × 10 mL
White blood cells (WBCs)	4000–10,000 mm³
Neutrophils	Adult: 48%–73%
	Child: 30%–60%
Lymphocytes	Adult: 18%–48%
	Child: 25%–50%
Monocytes	0%–9%
Eosinophil	0%–5%
Basophil	0–2%
Hemoglobin (Hgb)	Males: 13–18 g/dL
	Females: 12–16 g/dL
Hematocrit (Hct)	Males: 40%–54%
	Females: 37%–47%

Coagulation

Platelet	130,000–400,000 mL
Prothrombin time (PT)	10–14 sec
Partial thromboplastin time (PTT)	30–45 sec
Thrombin time (TT)	Control ±5 sec
Fibrinogen split products (FSP)	Negative reaction at >1:4 dilution
Iron or ferritin (Fe) (deficiency)	0–20 ng/mL
Reticulocyte count	0.5–1.5% of RBC

Laboratory Values—cont'd	
Laboratory Test	**Reference Range**

Blood Chemistry

Sodium (Na^+)	135–145 mEq/L
Potassium (K^+)	3.5–5.5 mEq/L
Chloride (Cl^-)	95–112 mEq/L
Anion gap	4–14 mEq/L
Carbon dioxide (CO_2)	24–32 mEq/L
Blood urea nitrogen (BUN)	7–25 mg/dL
Creatinine (Cr)	0.7–1.3 mg/dL (males)
	0.6–1.2 mg/dL (females)
Glucose	70–110 mg/dL
Calcium (Ca^{++})	8.5–10.5 mg/dL
Magnesium (Mg)	1.3–2.1 mg/dL
Phosphorus	2.5–4.5 mg/dL
Osmolality	275–295 mOsm/kg

Hepatic Enzymes

Aspartate aminotransferase (AST)	0–42 U/L
Alanine aminotransferase (ALT)	0–48 U/L
Alkaline phosphatase (ALP)	Adult: 20–125 U/L
	Child: 40–400 U/L
Bilirubin: Direct	0–0.2 mg/dL
Bilirubin: Total	0–1.2 mg/lb
Amylase	50–150 U/L
Lipase	0–110 U/L

Urine Electrolytes

Sodium (Na^+)	40–220 mEq/L
Potassium (K^+)	25–125 mEq/L
Chloride (Cl^-)	110–250 mEq/L

Continued

Laboratory Values—cont'd	
Laboratory Test	**Reference Range**

Lipids

Cholesterol	120–240 mg/dL
Low density lipoprotein (LDL)	62–130 mg/dL
High density lipoprotein (HDL)	35–135 mg/dL
Triglycerides	0–200 mg/dL
Cholesterol:LDL ratio	1:6–1:4.5

Thyroid

Thyroxine (T4)	4–12 µg/dL
Triiodothyronine (T3) uptake	27–47%
Thyroid-stimulating hormone (TSH)	0.5–6 milU/L

Cardiac Enzymes

Creatine phosphokinase (CK) Levels rise 4 to 8 hours after an acute myocardial infarction (MI), peaking at 16 to 30 hours and returning to baseline within 4 days (25–200 U/L; 32–150 U/L)

CK-MB CK isoenzyme Increases 6 to 10 hours after an acute MI, peaks in 24 hours, and remains elevated for up to 72 hours

<12 IU/L if total CK is <400 IU/L

<3.5% of total CK if total CK is >400 IU/L

Lactate dehydrogenase (LDH) Increases 2 to 5 days after an MI; the elevation can last 10 days (140–280 U/L)

*Averages may vary per facility.

Acid–Base Imbalances

Clinical Manifestations

Acidosis	Alkalosis

Respiratory Manifestations

Causes

Carbonic excess, pneumonia, hyperventilation, obesity	Carbonic deficit, anxiety, fear, hyperventilation, anemia, asthma

Signs and Symptoms

Confusion or CNS depression	Unconsciousness (late sign)

Laboratory Values

pH, 7.25 (low)	pH, 7.52 (high)
$PaCO_2$, 60 mm Hg (high)	$PaCO_2$, 31 mm Hg (low)
Bicarbonate, normal	Bicarbonate normal
$PaCO_2$, 60 mm Hg (acute)	PaO_2, 90 mm Hg (high)
PaO_2, 80 mm Hg (chronic)	

Metabolic Manifestations

Causes

Bicarbonate deficit, ketoacidosis, starvation, shock, diarrhea, renal failure	Bicarbonate excess, Cushing syndrome, hypokalemia, hypercalcemia, excessive vomiting, diuretics

Continued

Acid–Base Imbalances—cont'd	

Clinical Manifestations

Acidosis	Alkalosis
Signs and Symptoms	
Weakness, disorientation, coma	Respiratory depression, tetany, mental dullness
Laboratory Values	
pH <7.35	pH >7.45
Urine pH <6	Urine pH >7
$PaCO_2$, normal	$PaCO_2$, normal
K^+ >5	K^+ <3.5
Bicarbonate <21 mEq/L	Bicarbonate >28 mEq/L

CNS, central nervous system.

ARTERIAL BLOOD GASES

Acid–base balance (pH) Measures hydrogen concentration (7.35–7.45)

Oxygenation (PaO_2) Measures partial pressure of dissolved oxygen in the blood (80–100 mm Hg)

Saturation (SO_2) Measures percentage of oxygen to hemoglobin (95–98%)

Ventilation ($PaCO_2$) Measures partial pressure of carbon dioxide (38–45 mm Hg)

Nursing Interventions

Preparation Cleanse the area over the artery per organizational policy. Collect an arterial blood gas (ABG) per organizational policy.

Post-ABG The sample needs to go to the laboratory immediately. Some facilities may require an advance call to the laboratory before an ABG test specimen can be sent.

ELECTROLYTE IMBALANCES
Clinical Manifestations
Hyponatremia (less than 135 mEq/L)
Signs and symptoms Fatigue; abdominal cramps; diarrhea; weakness; hypotension; cool, clammy skin.
Causes Overhydration, kidney disease, diarrhea, syndrome of inappropriate antidiuretic hormone secretion (SIADH)

Hypernatremia (greater than 145 mEq/L)
Signs and symptoms Thirst; dry, sticky mucous membranes; dry tongue and skin; flushed skin; increased body temperature
Causes Dehydration, starvation

Hypokalemia (less than 3.5 mEq/L)
Signs and symptoms Weakness, fatigue, anorexia, abdominal distention, arrhythmias, decreased bowel sounds
Causes Diarrhea, diuretics, alkalosis, polyuria

Hyperkalemia (greater than 5 mEq/L)
Signs and symptoms Anxiety, arrhythmias, increased bowel sounds
Causes Burns, renal failure, dehydration, acidosis

Hypocalcemia (less than 8.3 mEq/L)
Signs and symptoms Abdominal cramps, tingling, muscle spasms, convulsions; assess magnesium level

Causes Parathyroid dysfunction, vitamin D deficiency, pancreatitis.

Hypercalcemia (greater than 10 mEq/L)
Signs and symptoms Deep bone pain, nausea, vomiting, constipation; assess magnesium level
Causes Parathyroid tumor, bone cancer or metastasis, osteoporosis

Hypomagnesemia (less than 1.3 mEq/L)
Signs and symptoms Tremors, muscle cramps, tachycardia, hypertension, confusion; assess calcium level
Causes Parathyroid dysfunction, cancer, chemotherapy, polyuria

Hypermagnesemia (greater than 2.5 mEq/L)
Signs and symptoms Lethargy, respiratory difficulty, coma; assess calcium level
Causes Parathyroid dysfunction, renal failure

Hypochloremia (or Hypochloremia)
(less than 96 mEq/L)
Signs and symptoms Fatigue, weakness, dizziness
Causes Loss of fluid, severe vomiting or diarrhea, prolonged diuretic or laxative use

Hyperchloremia (or Hyperchloremia)
(greater than 108 mEq/L)
Signs and symptoms Thirst; dry mucous membranes, tongue, and skin
Causes High sodium level, kidney failure, diabetes insipidus, diabetic coma

Hypophosphatemia (less than 2.2 mEq/L)
Signs and symptoms Nausea, bone and joint pain, constipation
Causes After stomach surgery, lack of vitamin D, high calcium levels, kidney damage, several endocrine disorders

Hyperphosphatemia (greater than 4.8 mEq/L)
Signs and symptoms Abdominal cramps, numbness and tingling
Causes Excess dairy intake, increased vitamin D, low calcium levels, kidney failure, tumor lysis syndrome

FLUID VOLUME IMBALANCES
Fluid Volume Deficit (Hypovolemia)
Signs and symptoms Hypotension, weight loss, decreased tearing or saliva, dry skin or mouth, oliguria, increased pulse or respirations, increased specific gravity of urine, increased serum sodium levels
Causes Dehydration, insufficient fluid intake, diuretics, sweating or polyuria, excessive tube feedings leading to diarrhea

Fluid Volume Excess (Hypervolemia)
Signs and symptoms Edema, puffy face or eyelids, ascites, rales or wheezes in lungs, bounding pulse, hypertension, sudden weight gain, decreased serum sodium levels
Causes Overhydration, renal failure, congestive heart failure

Common Fluid Volumes*

Small glass of water: 200 mL

Small bowl of soup: 180 mL

Water pitcher: 1 L

Ice cream: 120 mL

Juice: 120 mL

Teapot: 240 mL

Gelatin: 120 mL

Medium cup: 30 mL

Common Intravenous Solutions

Normal saline (NS): 0.9% saline

5% Dextrose in water (D_5W)

5% Dextrose in 0.9% saline (D_5NS)

5% Dextrose in 0.45% saline ($D_5 \frac{1}{2} NS$)

Lactated Ringer's solution ($NaCl$, K^+, Ca^{++}, lactic acid)

---

*Volumes may vary per institution.

	Drugs Affecting Hemostasis			
Medication	Drug Class	Peak Time	Duration	Half-Life
Alteplase	Thrombolytic	5–10 min	2–3 hr	5 min
Anistreplase	Thrombolytic	45 min	4–6 hr	70–120 min
Aspirin	Antiplatelet	15 min–2 hr	4–6 hr	15–30 min
Dalteparin	Anticoagulant	3–5 hr	12 hr	3.5 hr
Dipyridamole	Antiplatelet	75 min (PO)	3–4 hr	10 hr
		6.5 min (IV)	30 min	10 hr
Enoxaparin	Anticoagulant	3–5 hr	12 hr	4.5 hr
Heparin	Anticoagulant	2–4 hr (SC)	8–12 hr	1–2 hr
		5–10 (min) (IM)	2–6 hr	1–2 hr
Ibuprofen	NSAID, antiplatelet	1–2 hr	4–6 hr	1.8–2 hr
Ketorolac	NSAID, antiplatelet	30–60 min (PO)	4–6 hr	2–8 hr
		30–90 min (IM)	4–8 hr	5–6 hr

Continued

Drugs Affecting Hemostasis—cont'd				
Medication	Drug Class	Peak Time	Duration	Half-Life
Pentoxifylline	Antiplatelet	1–4 hr	Unknown	0.8–1.6 hr
Plavix	Antiplatelet	1 hr	Unknown	8 hr
Reteplase	Thrombolytic	5–10 min	Unknown	13–16 min
Streptokinase	Thrombolytic	30–60 min	4–12 hr	23 min
Sulfinpyrazone	Antiplatelet	1–2 hr	4–6 hr	4hr
Ticlopidine	Antiplatelet	2 hr	14–21 days	12.6 hr single dose / 4–5 days multidose
Urokinase	Thrombolytic	End of infusion	12 hr	20 min
Warfarin	Anticoagulant	0.5–3 days	2–5 days	0.5–3 days

IM, intramuscular; IV, intravenous; NSAID, nonsteroidal antiinflammatory drug; PO, oral; SC, subcutaneous.
Data from *Drug facts & comparisons*, St. Louis, 2002, Facts & Comparisons; *Physicians' desk reference*, ed 54, Montvale, NJ, 2000, Medical Economics.

DIAGNOSTIC TESTS

Angiography Records cardiac pressures, function, and output (Patient may need special postprocedure vital signs taken.)

Antinuclear antibody (ANA) A group of antibodies used to diagnose lupus (SLE)

Arterial blood gases Measurements of arterial blood pH, PO_2, $PaCO_2$, and bicarbonate (Blood sample needs to be kept on ice.)

Arteriography Radiographic examination with injections of dye used to locate occlusions (Patient may need special postprocedure vital signs taken.)

Arthrography Radiographic examination of the bones

Arthroscopy Procedure that allows examination of the joint

Barium study Radiographic examination to locate polyps, tumors, or other colon problems (Barium needs to be removed after procedure.)

Barium swallow Detects esophageal narrowing, varices, strictures, or tumors (Barium needs to be removed after procedure.)

Biopsy Removal of specific tissue (Assess patient for pain after procedure.)

Blood tests See section on laboratory values for normal values

Bone densitometry Test to determine bone mineral content and density; used to diagnose osteoporosis

Bone marrow biopsy Examination of a piece of tissue from bone marrow (Assess patient for pain after procedure.)

Bone scan Radioisotope used to locate tumors or other bone disorders (Patient must be able to lie flat.)

Brain scan Radioisotope used to locate tumors, strokes, or seizure disorders (Patient must be able to lie flat.)

Bronchoscopy Inspection of the larynx, trachea, and bronchi with flexible scope (Patient may need sedation.)

Cardiac catheterization Uses dye to visualize the heart's arteries (Patient may need special postprocedure vital signs taken.)

Chest radiographs Used to look for pneumonia, cancer, and other diseases of the lung

Cholangiography Radiographic examination of the biliary ducts

Cholecystography Radiographic examination of the gallbladder

Colonoscopy Uses flexible scope to view colon (Patient may need to be sedated.)

Colposcopy Examination of the cervix and vagina

Computed tomography (CT) scan Three-dimensional radiography (Patient must be able to lie flat.)

Culdoscopy Flexible tube used to view pelvic organs

Culture and sensitivity Determines source and type of bacteria

Cystoscopy Direct visualization of bladder with cystoscope

Dilatation and curettage Dilatation of the cervix followed by endometrial cleansing (done in surgery)

Doppler Ultrasonography used to show venous or arterial patency

Echocardiography Ultrasonography that records structure and functions of the heart

Electrocardiography Records electrical impulses generated by the heart

Electroencephalography (EEG) Records electrical activity of the brain (Patient should be resting.)

Electromyography (EMG) Records electrical activity of the muscles

Endoscopy Inspection of upper gastrointestinal (GI) tract with flexible scope (Patient may need to be sedated.)

Endoscopic retrograde cholangiopancreatography (ERCP) Radiographic examination of the gallbladder and pancreas

Exercise stress test Recording of the heart rate, activity, and blood pressure while the body is at work

Fluoroscopy Radiographic examination with picture displayed on television monitor

GI series Radiographic examination using barium to locate ulcers (Barium must be removed after procedure.)

Glucose tolerance test (GTT) Determines ability to tolerate an oral glucose load; used to establish diabetes

Hemoccult Detects blood in stool, emesis, and elsewhere

Holter monitor Checks and records irregular heart rates and rhythms (generally over a 24-hr period)

Intravenous pyelography (IVP) Radiographic examination of the kidneys after dye injection

KUB Radiographic examination of the kidneys, ureter, and bladder

Laparoscopy Abdominal examination with a flexible scope

Lumbar puncture Sampling of spinal fluid, often called a spinal tap (can be done bedside)

Magnetic resonance imaging (MRI) Three-dimensional radiograph similar to CT scan

Mammography Radiographic examination of the breast

Myelography Injection of dye into subarachnoid space to view brain and spinal cord

Oximetry Method to monitor arterial blood saturation

Pap smear Detects cervical cancer

Proctoscopy Inspection of lower colon with flexible scope (Patient may need to be sedated.)

Pulmonary function test (PFT) Measures lung capacity and volume to detect problems

Pyelography Radiographic examination of kidneys

Sigmoidoscopy Inspection of lower colon with flexible scope (Patient may need to be sedated.)

Small bowel follow-through (SBFT) Done in addition to a GI series

Spinal tap See lumbar puncture

Thallium Radionuclear dye used to assess heart functions

Titer A blood test to determine the presence of antibodies

Tuberculin skin test Test for tuberculosis using tuberculin purified protein derivative (PPD)

Ultrasonography Reflection of sound waves

Urine tests See Chapter 14

Venography Radiographic examination used to locate a thrombus in a vein

CHAPTER 17

Surgical Nursing Care

For an in-depth study of surgical nursing care, consult the following publications:

Lewis SM, et al: *Medical-surgical nursing*, ed 8, St. Louis, 2011, Mosby.

Nugent P, Green J, Hellmer Saul MA, Pelikan P: *Mosby's comprehensive review of nursing for the NCLEX-RN examination*, ed 20, St. Louis, 2012, Mosby.

Patton K, Thibodeau G: *Structure and function of the human body*, ed 14, St. Louis, 2012, Mosby.

Potter PA, Perry AG, Stockert PA, Hall A: *Fundamentals of nursing,* ed 8, St. Louis, 2013, Mosby.

Weilitz P, Potter PA: *Pocket guide for health assessment*, ed 6, St. Louis, 2007, Mosby.

NURSING CARE BEFORE SURGERY

Teaching

Include the following information:

Smoking or drinking restrictions before surgery

Dietary or fluid restrictions before surgery

Review of surgical procedure

Postoperative deep breathing, positioning, and range of motion exercises

Postoperative pain and pain relief measures available

Postoperative activity or dietary restrictions

Postoperative dressing procedures

Review of drains, nasogastric, catheter, and intravenous (IV) lines that may be inserted during surgery

History

Include the following information:

Chief complaint or reason for surgery

Prior surgeries and responses or impressions

Drug allergies

Physical limitations such as vision or hearing problems, limps, or paralysis

History of smoking and drinking

Last drink or food intake

Medications and the last time taken

Nonprescription or recreational drug use and when taken last

History of strokes, heart attacks, seizures, diabetes, and thyroid or adrenal disease

Concerns, questions, or special requests

Significant other and where he or she can be reached after surgery

Checklist

Include the following information:

Signed consent form in front of the chart

List of clothes and valuables and their placement in a safe place

Record of vital signs and last time voided

List of prostheses such as dentures and limbs removed

List of preoperative medications and when administered

Review of preoperative laboratory values and tests

Preoperative surgical scrubbing

Review of Body Systems

Note any problems, including the following:

Cardiac Arrhythmia, edema, cyanosis, chest pain, hypertension, murmur, heart rate, blood pressure

Respiratory Cough, shortness of breath, dyspnea, wheezing, orthopnea, orthostasis, diminished sounds, rate, depth

Neurologic Headaches, dizziness, ringing in ears, gait, reflexes, muscle strength, emotions

Gastrointestinal Nausea, vomiting, weight gain or loss, ulcers, Crohn disease or ulcerative colitis, devices

Genitourinary Urgency, frequency, retention, urinary tract infections, need for Foley catheter or other devices

Skin Bruising, open sores, rashes, signs of infection, general condition

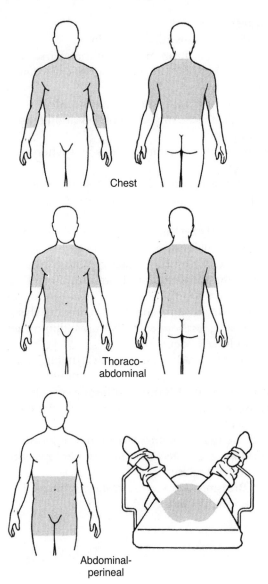

Chest

Thoraco-
abdominal

Abdominal-
perineal

FIGURE 17-1 Surgical skin preparations.

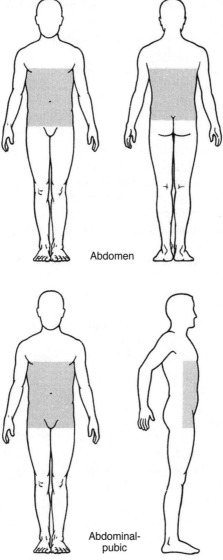

Abdomen

Abdominal-
pubic

FIGURE 17-2 Surgical skin preparations.

NURSING CARE AFTER SURGERY
Objectives
Provide a safe environment for the patient.

Monitor the patient's condition.

Recognize potential complications.

Prevent complications.

Information Needed*
Type of surgery and anesthetic

Findings and results of the surgery

Any complications during the surgery

Transfusions given during surgery

Current respiratory condition of the patient

Current cardiac and circulatory condition of the patient

Types and number of incisions, drains, tubes, and IV lines

Current vital signs and when they need to be taken next

Current laboratory values and when specimens need to be drawn next

Dressing location, condition, and changes (the first change is generally done by the surgeon)

Neurologic status and need for future neurologic checks

Time, frequency, and route of administration of pain medications

Additional postoperative orders

Notify any family or significant others waiting for the patient

---

*Can be found in the patient's chart.

CARE OF BODY SYSTEMS AFTER SURGERY

Cardiac

Possibility of hemorrhage, shock, embolism, thrombosis

Monitor blood pressure, heart rate, rhythm, quality.

Check for Homans sign, leg tenderness, leg edema.

Check capillary refill, hemorrhage, shock, pedal pulses.

Pulmonary

Possibility of obstruction, atelectasis, pneumonia

Turn patient every 1 to 2 hours unless contraindicated.

Have patient cough and deep breathe using pillows to splint incisions every 1 to 2 hours.

Assess lungs for rales, rhonchi, or wheezes.

Check oxygen saturation per policy protocol or with each check of vital signs.

Perform oral or deep suction as needed.

Have patient use incentive spirometer as ordered every 1 to 2 hours.

Use humidification to ease breathing and chest therapy if ordered.

Ensure adequate hydration to help thin secretions and postural drainage to drain secretions.

Assess for adequate pain relief to help breathing.

Neurologic

Perform neurologic and reflex checks as needed.

Assess orientation, level of consciousness, and pain control as needed.

Assess for restlessness, fatigue, and anxiety.

Explain the need for the procedure to the patient.

Genitourinary

Assess for adequate fluid intake and output and for bladder distention.

Assess the need for and care of Foley catheter or need for straight catheterization.

Gastrointestinal

Assess bowel sounds for possible ileus (indicated by no sounds).

Assess for nausea, vomiting, distended abdomen, and gas pains.

Skin

Assess wound for drainage and signs of infection.

Assess for skin breakdown.

Types of Dressings	
Name	**Uses**
Absorbent	Drains wound (increases evaporation)
Antiseptic	Prevents infection
Dry	With wound with little or no drainage
Hot and moist	Promotes wound healing by second or third intention; increases blood supply to wound
Occlusive	Prevents invasion of bacteria
Protective	Protects wound from injury
Wet to damp	Dressing removed before wound dries
Wet to dry	With open wound that has necrotic tissue; wound with greatest drainage
Wet to wet	With wound that needs to be kept very moist

COMMON SURGICAL PROCEDURES*

Anastomosis Creation of a passage between two vessels

Angiectomy or angioplasty Removal or repair of a vessel

Aortotomy Incision into the aorta

Arteriectomy or arterioplasty Removal or repair of an artery

Arthrectomy or arthroplasty Removal or repair of a joint

Atriotomy Incision into an atrium of heart

Biopsy Incision to remove a tissue sample

Bronchotomy or bronchoplasty Incision into repair of bronchus

Cholecystectomy Removal of the gallbladder

Choledochectomy Removal of a portion of the common bile duct

Colectomy Partial removal of the colon

Coronary artery bypass graft (CABG) A large vein from the body is removed and sutured to either side of an obstructed coronary artery

Craniectomy or cranioplasty Removal or repair of a portion of the skull

Cystectomy or cystoplasty Removal or repair of the bladder

Dermabrasion Surgical removal of epidermis or a portion of the dermis

Embolization Suturing or sealing of a vessel

Esophagectomy or esophagoplasty Removal or repair of the esophagus

Fasciectomy or fascioplasty Removal or repair of the fascia

Gastrectomy or gastroplasty Removal or repair of the stomach

---

*Refer to sections on prefixes and suffixes to build your surgical vocabulary.

Graft Surgical replacement of tissue, skin, or muscle

Hysterectomy Removal of the uterus

Laminectomy Removal of the posterior arch of a vertebra

Laryngectomy or laryngoplasty Removal or repair of the larynx

Lymphangiectomy or lymphangioplasty Removal or repair of a lymph vessel

Mastectomy or mastopexy Removal or reduction of a breast

Myectomy or myoplasty Removal or repair of an ovary

Nephrectomy Removal of a kidney

Oophorectomy or oophoroplasty Removal or repair of a testicle

Orchiectomy or orchioplasty Removal or repair of a testicle

Osteoclasis Reconstruction of a fractured bone

Percutaneous transluminal coronary angioplasty (PTCA) A balloon procedure used to push an obstruction against a vessel wall to allow blood to flow through

Pericardiectomy Removal of the pericardium

Phlebectomy or phleboplasty Removal or repair of a vein

Pneumonectomy Removal of a lung

Radical mastectomy Removal of a breast, pectorals, lymph nodes, and skin

Rhinoplasty Plastic repair of the nose

Splenotomy or splenorrhaphy Incision into or repair of the spleen

Thoracoplasty Removal of a rib to allow collapse of the lungs

Valvulotomy or valvuloplasty Incision into or repair of a valve

RED BLOOD CELL TRANSFUSIONS

Typing Selecting the ABO blood type and Rh
 antigen factor of a person's blood (other
 antigens can also affect transfusion
 compatibility)

Cross-matching Mixing the recipient's serum with
 the donor's red blood cells in a saline solution; if
 no agglutination occurs, the blood may be safely
 given

Transfusion Compatibility Table		
Blood Type	**Can Generally Donate to**	**Can Generally Receive From**
A–	A–, A+	A–, O–
B–	B–, B+	B–, O–
AB–	AB–, AB+	AB–, A–, B–, O
A+	A+	A+, A–, O+, O–
B+	B+	B+, B–, O+, O–
AB+	AB+	All blood types
O–	All blood types	O–
O+	O+, A+, B+, AB+	O+, O–

Before Administering Blood to a Patient

Check facility's policy on infusing blood products.
Check the patient's ID band for proper
 identification.
Check the patient's blood type and Rh antigen.
Get the blood from blood bank only when ready to
 infuse.

Compare the patient's blood type with the type of blood to be infused.

Two people should check and co-sign blood.

Start infusion of blood with normal saline solution.

Administer blood at a slower rate for the first 15 minutes. Blood should be infused within 4 hours.

Use appropriate blood tubing and needles (may vary per facility).

Document action on appropriate flow sheets (may vary per facility).

Instruct patient to report *any* discomfort (blood reactions).

Special vital signs are needed (may vary per facility).

Some facilities may medicate the patient with acetaminophen or diphenhydramine (Benadryl) before infusion.

Blood Reactions

Possible reactions include difficulty breathing, wheezing, tachypnea, fever, tachycardia, change in blood pressure, chest pain, disorientation, rash, or hives. *If a reaction begins, stop the infusion.* Begin a normal saline flush to keep the IV line open and administer prescribed antihistamines. Notify a physician, recheck blood, retype, and cross-match. *Do not* discard the blood—the laboratory may want to analyze it for the cause of the reaction. The physician may require a urine sample from the patient.

BLOOD TRANSFUSION ALTERNATIVES

Considerations for patients who may refuse blood transfusions based on cultural or religious reasons include:

Volume Expanders
Crystalloid Ringer's lactate, normal saline, hypertonic saline
Colloids Dextran, gelatin, hetastarch
Perfluorochemicals Fluosol DA-20

Hemostatic Agents for Bleeding or Clotting Problems
Topical—Avitene, Gelfoam, Oxycel, Surgicel
Injectable—Desmopressin, tranexamic acid, ε-aminocaproic acid, vitamin K

Techniques and Agents for Managing Anemia
Oxygen support
Maintain intravascular volume
Nutritional support
Iron
Dextran (Imferon)
Folic acid
Vitamin B_{12}
Erythropoietin
Granulocyte colony-stimulating factor (GCSF)
Perfluorocarbon solutions

Techniques to Limit Blood Loss During Surgery
Hypotensive anesthesia
Induced hypothermia
Intraoperative blood salvage
Intraoperative or hypervolemia hemodilution
Reduce blood flow to skin
Mechanical occlusion of bleeding vessels
Meticulous hemostasis

Techniques That Can Limit Blood Sampling
Transcutaneous pulse oximeter
Pulse oximeter
Pediatric microsampling
Planning ahead with multiple tests per sample

Techniques to Locate and Arrest Internal Bleeding

Electrocautery
Laser surgery
Argon beam coagulator
Endoscope
Gamma knife radiosurgery
Embolization

CHAPTER 18

Patient Safety

Admission Safety (p. 314)
Ongoing Safety (p. 314)
Special Patient Situations (p. 315)
The Confused Patient (p. 317)
Common Psychiatric Disorders (p. 321)
Common Psychiatric Tests (p. 322)
Treatment Methods (p. 322)
Emergencies (p. 323)

For an in-depth study of patient safety, consult
the following publications:

Lewis SM, et al: *Medical-surgical nursing*, ed 8, St. Louis, 2011, Mosby.
Lueckenotte AB: *Pocket guide to gerontologic assessment*, ed 3, St. Louis, 1998, Mosby.
Nugent P, Green J, Hellmer Saul MA, Pelikan P: *Mosby's comprehensive review of nursing for the NCLEX-RN examination*, ed 20, St. Louis, 2012, Mosby.
Potter PA, Perry AG, Stockert PA, Hall A: *Fundamentals of nursing,* ed 8, St. Louis, 2013, Mosby.
Weilitz P, Potter PA: *Pocket guide for health assessment*, ed 6, St. Louis, 2007, Mosby.

ADMISSION SAFETY

When a patient is admitted to the hospital or nursing home, it is important that the patient is aware of all equipment located in his or her room. This can prevent accidents and make the stay in the hospital or nursing home safer. Point out the following items on admission: call light or bell, room lights, bathroom, bathroom lights, nurses' station, side rails, and room number.

Make sure that all equipment is working properly.

ONGOING SAFETY

To ensure ongoing safety, take the following precautions:

Clear the patient's room of excess debris.

No furniture should block the doorway to the patient's room.

Immediately clean up any water or other liquid spills on the floor.

Do not leave needles or other sharp items near the patient.

Remove unmarked bottles and syringes from patient's room.

Label all intravenous and central lines, and nasogastric, gastrostomy, and jejunostomy tubes.

Check all electrical equipment for proper functioning and condition.

Double check all medications before giving them to the patient, referring to the 10 patient rights.

Double check the patient's identification ID bracelet before giving medications, performing any procedures, and transferring the patient to another department for tests, another unit, surgery, or therapy appointments.

SPECIAL PATIENT SITUATIONS
Hospitalized patients with the following problems may require additional safety measures:

Alcohol Withdrawal
Signs and Symptoms. Confusion, sweating, pallor, palpitations, hypotension, seizures, coma. Protocols may vary by facility.

Withdrawal protocols may include seizure precautions, keeping the side rails up and padded, taking vital signs frequently (every 30–60 minutes or per hospital protocol), and close observation. Provide a safe environment. Perform neurologic, memory, and orientation checks. Document any withdrawal activity and actions taken.

Bleeding or Hemorrhage
Locate the source of the bleeding. Apply direct pressure with a clean drape. Call for assistance but stay with the patient. Assess for early signs of shock such as a change in sensorium and later signs of shock such as hypotension; pale skin; and a rapid, weak pulse.
Prevention. Closely supervise confused or heavily medicated patients and patients just returning from surgery. Make sure surgical dressings are secure. Encourage patients to call for assistance if bleeding begins. Document any bleeding and actions taken.

Choking
Follow standard Heimlich maneuver guidelines.
Prevention. Closely supervise confused and heavily medicated patients. Make sure patients are sitting up or are placed in high Fowler's position when eating. Encourage the use of the call lights. Assess the patient's ability to chew and swallow.

Order a diet appropriate to the patient's eating ability. Document any choking situations and actions taken.

Drug Reactions

Assess for difficulty breathing, wheezing, tearing, palpitations, skin rash, pruritus, nausea or vomiting, rhinitis, diarrhea, and a change in mood or mental status. *These are general drug reactions, not the side effects of specific drugs. Immediately report all drug reactions.*

Prevention. Closely supervise confused and heavily medicated patients and patients who are taking medications for the first time. Encourage the use of the call lights if any of the signs of a drug reaction occur. *Know your patient's drug allergies.* Document all drug reactions and actions taken.

Syncope and Common Causes

Neurologic Vertebrobasilar transient ischemic attacks, subclavian steal syndrome, hydrocephalus

Metabolic Hypoxia, hyperventilation, hypoglycemia

Cardiac Orthostatic hypotension, vasovagal reaction or syncope

Vasomotor Obstructive lesions, arrhythmias

Assess for dizziness, lightheadedness, visual blurring or any visual or hearing changes, weakness, apprehension, nausea, sweating, blood pressure, and pulse

Prevention or intervention *Stay with the patient.* Help patient sit or lower to the chair, bed or floor. Protect patient's head *at all times. Call for help.* Elevate the legs, assess vital signs, use ammonia (if needed), help the patient sit up slowly when he or she is ready, and document per organizational policy.

THE CONFUSED PATIENT

Assess for the source of the confusion. Possible sources include age, medications, disease, and infection. Confused patients may be at risk for falls.

Falls

Assess for the patient's ability to ambulate, environment, mental status, medications.
Prevention. Closely supervise confused and heavily medicated patients, encourage the use of call lights or the use of night lights, raise side rails, post sign alerting others of the possibility of falls, lock wheelchair, use gait belts, encourage the patient to use grab bars or side rails, avoid water and other liquid spills, and use nonskid footwear.

Falls Assessment Checklist

One or more of the following items can place a person at risk for falls:

___ Older than 70 years old	___ Weak
___ Hearing or visual loss	___ Urinary frequency
___ Disoriented or confused	___ Agitated
___ History of falls	
	___ Uses cane or walker
___ Does not speak or understand English	___ Psychotropic drug use
___ Diuretic use	___ Cardiac drug use
___ Electrolyte imbalance	___ Hypotensive
___ Cardiac disease	___ Neurologic disease
___ Recent myocardial infarction	___ Peripheral vascular disease
___ Uncontrolled diabetes	___ Recent cerebrovascular accident

Restraints
When to Use
- To prevent injury
- To restrict movement
- To immobilize a body part
- To prevent harm to self or others

Restraints should be used only when all other methods of keeping a patient safe have been tried.

Types of Restraints
Jackets or vests, belts, mittens, wrist or ankle, crib net, elbow

Guidelines
- Obtain physician's order and follow facility protocol.
- Explain purpose to patient; check circulation every 30 minutes.
- Release temporarily (once per hour).
- Provide range of motion.
- Document need and examination schedule.
- Report problems and tolerance; provide emotional support.

Never secure restraints to the side rails or the nonstationary portion of the main frame of the bed.

Complications
- Skin breakdown (pad bony areas)
- Nerve damage (do not overtighten; release often)
- Circulatory impairment (check for problems often; provide range of motion)
- Death (from inadequate or improper use)

Prevention
- Keep the side rails up when you are not with the patient.
- Monitor vital signs and the patient's drug doses and levels.
- Monitor the patient's electrolytes and neurologic status.
- Reorient patient to place and time as needed.
- Place call light in easy reach.
- Attend closely to personal care needs.
- Encourage family, friends, and clergy to visit often.

Comparison of Delirium and Dementia

Feature	Delirium	Dementia
Onset	Rapid, often at night	Usually insidious
Duration	Hours to weeks	Months to years
Course	Fluctuates over 24 hr Worse at night Lucid intervals	Relatively stable
Awareness	Always impaired	Usually normal
Alertness	Fluctuates	Usually normal
Orientation	Impaired; often will mistake people or places	May be intact May confabulate
Memory	Recent and immediate memory impaired	Recent and remote memory impaired
Thinking	Slow, accelerated, or dreamlike	Poor in abstraction Impoverished
Perception	Often misperceptions	Becomes absent
Sleep cycle	Disrupted at night Drowsiness during day	Fragmented sleep
Physical	Often sick	Often well at first

COMMON PSYCHIATRIC DISORDERS

Alcoholic psychosis A confused, disoriented state after intoxication

Anorexia nervosa An eating disorder; loss of appetite for food not explainable by disease

Anxiety disorder No mechanisms to block varying degrees of anxiety

Bulimia Disorder in which vomiting is self-induced after eating large amount of food

Conversion disorder Sensory or motor impairment in the absence of organic cause

Depression Feeling of hopelessness or sadness or loss of interest

Dissociative disorder Person escapes stress through memory or identity changes

Korsakoff syndrome Delirium or hallucinations often caused by chronic alcohol use

Mania Characterized by a state of extreme excitement

Manic-depressive Mood swing of very high to very low

Paranoia Delusions of persecution or of grandeur

Personality disorder Repetitive, irresponsible, and manipulative behaviors

Phobia A morbid fear or anxiety about an item or a place

Psychosis Loss of reality

Psychosomatic Person is limited in coping skills, which produces physical effects

Schizophrenia Profoundly withdrawn from reality, often with bizarre behaviors

COMMON PSYCHIATRIC TESTS

Beck Depression Inventory Self-report measure of feelings and attitudes

Brief Psychiatric Rating Scale Standardized rating scale for person older than 18 years of age

Rorschach Test Ten ink blots used to analyze thought processes

Thematic Apperception Test Unstructured set of pictures for which the patient makes up stories; to uncover conflict or to reveal needs

Wechsler Adult Intelligence Scale Verbal and cognitive test

TREATMENT METHODS

Antipsychotic drugs Antipsychotics and tranquilizers

Antidepressant drugs Tricyclics and monoamine oxidase (MAO) inhibitors

Antianxiety drugs Minor tranquilizers or propanediols and benzodiazepines

Behavior modification Rewards given to modify behavior

Behavior therapy Aversion therapy to modify behavior

Cognitive therapy Patient examines his or her own beliefs and attitudes

Electroconvulsive therapy Shock therapy given to the brain to induce a seizure

Insulin therapy Places patient in coma; used to treat patients with schizophrenia

Prefrontal lobotomy Frontal lobes of the brain are separated

Psychoanalytic therapy Therapy to gain insight into the origins of the condition

Psychotherapies Group therapy of psychiatric disorders

EMERGENCIES
Fire Safety
RACE—Rescue patients, **a**lert others/pull **a**larm, **c**ontain fire, **e**xtinguish fire. Know the facility's emergency telephone number. Know your location. Speak clearly. Know the facility's fire drill and evacuation plan. Close windows and doors. Turn off oxygen supply. All extinguishers are labeled A, B, C, or D according to the types of fires they are meant to extinguish. Some extinguishers can be used for more than one type of fire and are labeled with more than one letter. The types of fires the letters correspond to are:

A: Paper or wood
B: Liquid or gas
C: Electrical
D: Combustible metal

Any of the following emergencies may require cardiopulmonary resuscitation (CPR).

Heart Attack
Signs and symptoms Chest pain; shortness of breath; dyspnea; a squeezing, crushing, or heavy feeling in the chest; lightheadedness; pain in left arm or in the jaw; nausea
Intervention Calm the patient and turn on the call light. Begin oxygen at 2 L if nearby. Remain calm and stay with the patient until help arrives. Document symptoms and actions taken.

Pulmonary Embolism
Signs and symptoms Chest pain, shortness of breath, dyspnea, cyanosis, and possible death
Causes Immobility, deep vein thrombosis
Intervention Calm patient and turn on the call light. Begin oxygen at 2 L if nearby. Remain calm and stay with the patient until help arrives. Document symptoms and actions taken.

Prevention Elevate legs, use antiembolism stockings, dorsiflexion of foot, perform range of motion exercises, check Homans sign, perform coughing and deep breathing exercise, and administer low dosages of heparin as prescribed while patient is hospitalized. Do not massage lower legs.

Cardiac Arrest

Remain calm and turn on the call light. Begin CPR (follow standard guidelines) until more experienced staff arrives and takes over. Clear furniture from the room and ask family to move to waiting area. (Some facilities allow family to watch CPR activity.)

Seizures

Sign and Symptoms

Grand mal Total body stiffness, staring, jerking muscles

Petit mal Daydreaming, staring

Causes Neurologic disease, cancer, head injury, fever, or pregnancy-induced hypertension

Interventions Remain calm and turn on the call light. Ensure the patient's safety, lower the bed, and raise the side rails. Stay with the patient, time the seizure, and make sure the patient does not hit his or her head. Document seizure activity and actions taken.

Shock
Signs and Symptoms
Mild or early Warm, flushed skin, changes in orientation, widening pulse pressure

Moderate or mild Cool, clammy, pale skin; hypotension; narrowing pulse pressure; sweating; pallor; rapid pulse; decrease in urinary output

Severe or late All of the symptoms of moderate or mild shock plus irregular pulse, oliguria, shallow, rapid breathing, obtunded, or comatose

Causes Hemorrhage, infection, or hypovolemia

Intervention Monitor vital signs, assess orientation, and keep the patient warm. Record all symptoms and vital signs.

CHAPTER 19

Care of the Dying

For an in-depth study of death and dying, bereavement, and cultural and religious rituals, consult the following publications:

Giger JN: *Transcultural nursing: assessment and intervention*, ed 6, St. Louis, 2013, Mosby.

Husted GL, Husted JH: *Ethical decision making in nursing*, ed 2, St. Louis, 1995, Mosby.

Kübler-Ross E: *On death and dying*, New York, 1969, Collier Books.

Kübler-Ross E: *Questions and answers on death and dying*, New York, 1974, Collier Books.

STAGES OF DYING AND GRIEF
Denial
- Patient or family may refuse to accept the situation.
- Patient or family may not believe the diagnosis.
- Patient or family may seek second and third opinions.
- Patient or family may claim that the test results were wrong.
- Patient or family may claim that the tests were mixed up with those of someone else.
- Patient may sleep more or be overly talkative or cheerful.

Anger
- Patient or family may be hostile.
- Patient or family may have excessive demands.
- Patient may be withdrawn cold, or unemotional.
- Feelings may include envy, resentment, or rage.
- Patient may be angry at family for being well.
- Patient may be uncooperative or manipulative.
- This may be the time that patients are the hardest to care for but the time when they need us the most!

Bargaining
- Patient or family may promise to improve or change habits such as quit smoking, eat less, or exercise more.
- Bargaining may be intertwined with feelings of guilt.
- Bargains are often with the physicians or with God.

Depression

- Patient or family may speak of the upcoming loss.
- Patient or family may cry or weep often.
- Patient or family may want to be alone.

Acceptance

- Patient may exhibit a decreased interest in the surroundings.
- Patient may not want visitors during this time.
- Do not confuse acceptance with depression.
- There seems to be a calmness or peace about the patient.

INTERACTING WITH THE DYING PATIENT AND THE FAMILY

Interventions should be based on the stage of dying and grief.

Denial

This stage is used as a coping or protective function and should not be viewed as a bad quality. It can be a time when a patient or family can gather their thoughts, feelings, and strengths.

You should:
- Listen, listen, listen (remember, they may talk a lot).
- Get a sense of what they are worried about.
- Be honest with communications.
- Not give the patient false hope.
- Not argue with the patient or family.

Anger

This is often directed at caregivers; ensure that caregivers will not stop caring.

You should:
- Not take anger personally.
- Help family not to take anger personally.
- Visit the patient often and answer call lights promptly.
- Assist the family with much-needed breaks.

Bargaining

Because many of the bargains may be with a divine power, the period may pass unnoticed.

You should:
- Offer frequent chances for the patient or family to talk.
- Offer visits from clergy or other supports.

Depression
Some patients or families may not have a good outlet for their depression.

You should:
- Not force cheerful or important conversation.
- Allow the patient or family to voice concerns.
- Offer visits from clergy.
- Offer cultural or religious supports.

Acceptance
Patient may want to be alone and families may feel rejected.

You should:
- Encourage family to come often but for brief visits.
- Offer visits from clergy.
- Offer cultural or religious supports.

NURSING INTERVENTIONS WITH IMPENDING DEATH

Personal Care

- Good mouth care: keep mouth moist; do not use lemon swabs
- Skin care: use lotions, massage, good lip care
- Artificial tears if eyes are open
- Adequate pain control with medications, massage, and positioning
- Suctioning if there are increased secretions to ease breathing
- Clean and straighten linens often
- Change position of patient as needed to promote comfort
- Provide adequate hydration

Recognize Special Needs

- Encourage visits by clergy.
- Assess for the need for Last Rites, Holy Communion, or other ceremonies.
- Allow for religious music, holy books, and other supports.
- Allow time for the family or friends to pray.
- Encourage cultural or religious rituals or practices.

Prepare the Family

- Describe the physical changes that may be taking place as death approaches.
- Allow the family as much time as possible with the dying patient.
- Offer the family opportunities for cultural or religious rituals.
- Keep the family updated as to the time of approaching death.
- Be honest when telling the family about the impending death.
- Allow for sleep and hygiene needs of the family or friends.
- Allow the family or friends time to voice fears or concerns.
- Allow the family time for questions.
- Allow the family time for tears.

RELIGIOUS DEATH RITUALS

- **Buddhism** Belief in reincarnation; Last Rites and chanting at the bedside are encouraged.
- **Confucianism** Belief in reincarnation; burning incense and flowers are laid at the bedside to assist the spirit on its journey.
- **Eastern and Russian Orthodox** Last Rites must be conducted while the patient is still conscious.
- **Hindu** Patient may wish to be placed on the floor to be closer to the earth in death. Family is encouraged to wash and prepare the body. Chapters 2, 8, and 25 of the *Bhagavad-gita* and the holy book are read.
- **Jehovah's Witness** There are no special death rites; however, church elders may assist the family with final arrangements.
- **Judaism (Conservative and Orthodox)** The body is washed by the burial society and wrapped in white linen. No embalming or flowers are used. A cantor will assist the rabbi in the funeral. Burial should be done within 24 hours and should not be done on the Sabbath.
- **Judaism (Reform and Liberal)** No restrictions on the time or day of removal or burial.
- **Lutheran** May accept Holy Communion; Last Rites are optional.
- **Methodist and Baptist** May wish to invite religious clergy to be near at the time of death.
- **Mormon** Anointing of the sick and Communion are encouraged. Church elder may assist the family with arrangements. The body is washed by the relief society. If the person has been "through the temple," the person is dressed in white with a green apron.

- **Muslim** Chapter 36 of the *Qu'ran* is read to the patient. The family will encourage the patient to recite, "There is no god but Allah, and Mohammed is a messenger of Allah" before dying. The family will assist in washing the body and wrapping it in a white cloth.
- **Roman Catholic** Anointing of the sick and Holy Communion are encouraged. A rosary service the evening before the funeral is often done.
- **Shinto** All jewelry is to removed, and the body is washed and dressed in a white kimono.
- **Taoism** The family may wish to have a priest at the bedside at the time of death.

RELIGIOUS PRAYERS
Jewish Prayer on Behalf of the Sick

May God who blessed those who came before us in history and in life, heal _____ who is ill. May the Holy One have mercy upon _____; O Lord, reduce the pain and bind the wounds. Give skill to those who help in healing. And speedily restore _____ to perfect health, both spiritual and physical. Amen.

A Prayer for Quiet Confidence
The Very Reverend John Wallace Suter, Fourth Dean of Washington National Cathedral 1928
Book of Common Prayer

O God of peace, who hast taught us that in returning and rest we shall be saved, in quietness and confidence shall be our strength:

By the might of our Spirit lift us, we pray Thee, to Thy presence, where we may be still and know that Thou art God.

Through Jesus Christ our Lord, Amen.

A Litany for Preserving the Inner Self and the Earth
The Reverend Frederick Quinn, Chair of the Environment Committee of the Commission on Peace of the Diocese of Washington Cathedral

Lord of the universe, you placed the earth in our trust; help us to preserve it wisely. Help us to cherish ourselves upon this earth in all its mystery. Treasure its fragile beauty and honor its diversity; help us to turn from paths of selfishness and destruction; let all creation reflect God's wonder and all creatures, in their own voices, sing God's praise.

Muslim Prayer of Healing
(the Holy *Qu'ran,* Chapter Ii: 153–157)
O ye who believe! Seek help with patient perseverance and prayer; for God is with those who patiently persevere. And say not of those who are slain in the way nay, they are living, though ye perceive it not. Be sure we shall test you with something of fear and hunger, some loss in goods or lives or the fruits of your toil, but give glad tidings to those who patiently persevere. Who say, when afflicted with calamity: "To God we belong, and to Him is our return." They are those on whom descend blessings from God, and mercy, and they are the ones that receive guidance.

A Hindu Prayer for Healing the Body and Spirit
May the Supreme Lord of the Universe nourish the body so that I may have only auspicious words, that I may see only good things, that I may see the divinity in all things and everywhere experience the many forms of the One Supreme God: that all people on earth may be blessed.

LEGAL CONSIDERATIONS

Coroner's case Deaths in which the county coroner must be made aware, including deaths such as homicides, suicides, and suspicious or accidental deaths

Death certificate The legal document that identifies the date, time, and cause(s) of death

Documentation The date and time of death, along with the health care workers' final activities, should be noted in the patient's chart.

Do not resuscitate Because these words may have different meanings for different people, it should be clearly documented what the meaning is for each patient. Health care facilities should make sure that the wishes of the person and family are being carried out completely and correctly.

Establishing the time of death Absence of response to external stimuli, heart rate, respiration, and pupillary reflexes

Final disposition Final destination for the body. The hospital or county morgue or funeral home is generally the final disposition of the body.

Life-sustaining procedure Any medical procedure that in the judgment of the physician would only prolong the dying process

Living will A document that informs the physician that in the event of a terminal illness or injury the person wishes to have life-sustaining procedures stopped or withheld

Organ donations The law requires all hospitals that receive Medicare dollars to ask for organ donations on death.

Persistent vegetative state A condition of irreversible cessation of all functions of the cerebral cortex that results in a complete chronic and irreversible cessation of all cognitive functions. This condition must be documented by two physicians.

Postmortem or autopsy An examination conducted to determine the exact cause of death

Power of attorney for health care A legal document in which a person specifies another person to make his or her medical decisions in the event the person cannot

Pronouncement Certification as to the time of death. In most states, only a physician is responsible for this procedure.

CARE OF THE BODY IMMEDIATELY AFTER DEATH

If the family is *not* present at the time of death:

Assess for any special religious, cultural, or family instructions.

Review the facility's policies and procedure for preparation.

Assess for any legal limitations in preparing the body.

Wear gloves when preparing the body.

The body should be placed flat with the arms and legs straight.

The eyes and mouth should be closed.

Remove all intravenous lines, nasogastric tubes, Foley catheters, and so on.

Clean away any excretions and secretions.

Dress the body in a clean gown, if possible.

Remove all excess equipment and trash from room.

Set personal items (e.g., dentures, glasses) near the patient.

Pack up all other personal items.

Document your work in the patient's chart and wait for the family.

If the family is present at the time of death:

Allow the family time to be with their loved one.

Ask the family if there are any religious or cultural rituals that need to be honored.

Ask the family for time to prepare the body.

Allow the family to assist with the body if they wish.

Allow the family as much time as possible with the loved one.

Assist the family in packing up the belongings.

Assist the family with any paperwork.

Allow the family to call nonpresent family members, if needed.

Support the family in deciding on a funeral home or other arrangements.

After the family has gone, prepare the body for removal per the facility's protocol.

Document your work in the patient's chart.

General Guidelines for Autopsies, Burial Versus Cremation, and Organ Donations			
	Accepts Autopsies	Burial vs. Cremation	May Donate Organs
Agnostic	Yes	Both	Yes
Amish	Yes	Burial	Reluctant
Arab	Discouraged	Burial	Reluctant
Atheist	Yes	Both	Yes
Baha'i	Yes	Burial	Yes
Buddhist	Yes	Cremation	Yes
Cambodian	Yes	Both	Yes
Catholic (Orthodox)	Reluctant	Burial	Reluctant
Catholic (Roman)	Yes	Both	Yes
Chinese	Yes	Both	Yes
Christian	Yes	Both	Yes
Christian Scientist	Reluctant	Both	Reluctant
Eastern Orthodox	Reluctant	Burial	Yes

Continued

General Guidelines for Autopsies, Burial Versus Cremation, and Organ Donations—cont'd			
	Accepts Autopsies	Burial vs. Cremation	May Donate Organs
Filipino	Yes	Both	Yes
Gypsy	Reluctant	Burial	Reluctant
Hindu	Reluctant	Both	Yes
Hispanic	Yes	Both	Yes
Hmong	Yes	Both	Yes
Islamic	Reluctant	Burial	Reluctant
Japanese	Yes	Both	Yes
Jehovah's Witness	Reluctant	Both	Reluctant
Judaism (Hasidim)	Reluctant	Burial	Reluctant
Judaism (Orthodox)	Reluctant	Burial	Reluctant
Judaism (Reform)	Yes	Both	Yes
Korean	Yes	Both	Reluctant
Laotian	Yes	Both	Yes

Mennonite	Yes	Both	Yes
Mormon	Yes	Burial	Yes
Native American	Reluctant	Both	Reluctant
Quaker	Yes	Cremation	Yes
Russian Orthodox	Yes	Both	Yes
Seventh Day Adventist	Reluctant	Both	Yes
Shinto	No	Both	No
Sikhism	Reluctant	Stillborn: Burial All others: Cremated	Yes
Taoist	Yes	Both	Yes
Thai	Yes	Both	Yes
Vietnamese	Yes	Cremation	Yes

MULTIORGAN PROCUREMENT

Organs and Tissues That Can Be Donated

Organ Heart, lungs, liver, pancreas, kidneys, intestines

Bones and soft tissues Humerus, ribs, iliac crest, vertebrae, femur, tibia, fibula, tendons, ligaments, fascia lata

Other tissues Eyes, heart valves, skin, saphenous vein

Consent Hierarchy	Potential Donors
1. Signed donor card	1. Victims of cerebral trauma
2. Spouse	2. Trauma victims
3. Adult son or daughter	3. Some drug overdoses
4. Either parent	4. Primary brain tumors
5. Adult brother or sister	5. Anoxic brain damage
6. Grandparent	6. Cerebral or subarachnoid bleeds
7. Legal guardian	

Special Notes Regarding Procurement

Procuring an organ(s) is a surgical procedure that takes place in the operating room under sterile conditions.

When applicable, after the procurement, prosthetic replacement and proper suturing are completed to restore the body to its natural appearance.

Donating organs should not interfere with funeral arrangements or with the desire to have an open-casket funeral.

There is no cost to the donating family for the procurement or transplant procedure.

English-to-Spanish Translation Guide: Key Medical Questions

The following is a guide to help you complete the history and examination of Spanish-speaking patients. The first sets of questions are introductory and general ones used at the beginning of the examination. Questions for pain assessment follow. The rest is arranged by body system. Each system's section contains basic vocabulary, questions used for history taking, and instructions that would facilitate examination. The intent of this guide is to offer an array of questions and phrases from which the examiner can choose.

Hints for Pronunciation of Spanish Words
1. *h* is silent.
2. *j* is pronounced as h.
3. *ll* is pronounced as a *y* sound.
4. *r* is pronounced with a trilled sound, and *rr* is trilled even more.
5. *v* is pronounced with a *b* sound.
6. *i* and a *y* by itself are pronounced with a long e sound.
7. *qu* is pronounced as a *k* sound; *cu* is pronounced as a *qu* sound.
8. *e* is pronounced with a long *a* sound.
9. Accent marks over the vowel indicate the syllable that is to be stressed.

Introductory

I am _____.	Soy _____.
What is your name?	¿Cómo se llama usted?
I would like to examine you now.	Quisiera examinarlo(a) ahora.

General

How do you feel?	¿Cómo se siente?
Good	Bien
Bad	Mal
Do you feel better today?	¿Se siente mejor hoy?
Where do you work? (What is your profession or job?) (What do you do?)	¿Dónde trabaja? (¿Cuál es su profesión o trabajo?) (¿Qué hace usted?)
Are you allergic to anything?	¿Tiene usted algerias?
Medications, foods, insect bites?	¿Medicinas, alimentos, picaduras de insectos?
Do you take any medications?	¿Toma usted algunas medicinas?
Do you have any drug allergies?	¿Es usted alérgico (a) algún médicamento?
Do you have a history of heart disease?	¿Padece usted enfermedad?
diabetes?	del corazón?
epilepsy?	del diabetes?
bronchitis?	la epilepsia?
emphysema?	de bronquitis?
asthma?	de enfisema?
	de asma?

Pain

Have you any pain?	¿Tiene dolor?
Where is the pain?	¿Dónde está el dolor?

Do you have any pain here?	¿Tiene usted dolor aqui?
How severe is the pain?	¿Qué tan fuerte es el dolor?
Mild, moderate, sharp, or severe?	¿Ligero, moderado, agudo, severo?
What were you doing when the pain started?	¿Qué haciá usted cuando le comenzó el dolor?
Have you ever had this pain before?	¿Ha tenido este dolor antes?
	(¿Ha sido siempre así?)
Do you have a pain in your side?	¿Tiene usted dolor en el costado?
Is it worse now?	¿Está peor ahora?
Does it still pain you?	¿Le duele todavía?
Did you feel much pain at the time?	¿Sintió mucho dolor entonces?
Show me where.	Muéstreme dónde.
Does it hurt when I press here?	¿Le duele cuando aprieto aquí?

Head

Vocabulary

Head	La cabeza
Face	La cara

History

How does your head feel?	¿Cómo siente la cabeza?
Have you any pain in the head?	¿Le duele la cabeza?
Do you have headaches?	¿Tiene usted dolores de cabeza?
Do you have migraines?	¿Tiene usted migrañas?
What causes the headaches?	¿Qué le causa los dolores de cabeza?

Examination

Lift up your head.	Levante la cabeza.

Eyes
Vocabulary

Eye	El ojo

History

Have you had pain in your eyes?	¿Ha tenido dolor en los ojos?
Do you wear glasses?	¿Usa usted anteojos/gafas/lentes/espejuelos?
Do you wear contact lenses?	¿Usa usted lentes de contacto?
Can you see clearly?	¿Puede ver claramente?
Better at a distance?	¿Mejor a cierta distancia?
Do you sometimes see things double?	¿Ve las cosas doble algunas veces?
Do you see things through a mist?	¿Ve las cosas nubladas?
Were you exposed to anything that could have injured your eye?	¿Fue expuesto a cualquier cosa que pudiera haberle dañado el ojo?
Do your eyes water much?	¿Le lagrimean mucho los ojos?

Examination

Look up.	Mire para arriba.
Look down.	Mire para abajo.
Look toward your nose.	Mírese la nariz.
Look at me.	Míreme.
Tell me what number it is.	Digame qué número es ésta.
Tell me what letter it is.	Digame qué lera es éste.

Ears, Nose, and Throat

Vocabulary

Ears	Los oídos
Eardrum	El tímpano
Laryngitis	La laringitis
Lip	El labio
Mouth	La boca
Nose	La nariz
Tongue	La lengua

History

Do you have any hearing problems?	¿Tiene usted problemas de oir?
Do you use a hearing aid?	¿Usa usted un audífono?
Do you have ringing in the ears?	¿Le zumban los oídos?
Do you have allergies?	¿Tiene alergias?
Do you use dentures?	¿Usa usted dentadura postiza?
Do you have any loose teeth, removable bridges, or any prosthesis?	¿Tiene dientes flojos, dientes postizos, o cualquier prostesis?
Do you have a cold?	¿Tiene usted un resfriado/resfrío?
Do you have sore throats frequently?	¿Le duele la garganta con frecuencia?
Have you ever had a strep throat?	¿Ha tenido alguna vez infección de la garganta?

Examination

Open your mouth.	Abra la boca.
I want to take a throat culture. This will not hurt.	Quiero hacer un cultivo de la garganta. Esto no le va a doler.

Cardiovascular

Vocabulary

Heart	El corazón
Heart attack	El ataque al corazón
Heart disease	La enfermedad del corazón
Heart murmur	El soplo del corazón
High blood pressure	Presión alta

History

Have you ever had any chest pain?	¿Ha tenido alguna vez dolor de pecho?
Where?	¿Dónde?
Do you notice any irregularity of heart beat or any palpitations?	¿Nota cualquier latido o palpitación irregular?
Do you get short of breath?	¿Tiene usted problemas con la respiracion?
When?	¿Cuándo?
Do you take medicine for your heart?	¿Toma medicina para el corazón?
How often?	¿Con qué frecuencia?
Do you know if you have high blood pressure?	¿Sabe usted si tiene la presión alta?
Is there a history of hypertension in your family?	¿En su familia se encuentron varias personas con presión alta?
Are any of your limbs swollen?	¿Están hinchados algunos de sus miembros?
Hands, feet, legs?	¿Manos, pies, piernas?
How long have they been swollen like this?	¿Desde cuándo están hinchados así? (¿Qué tanto tiempo tiene usted con esta inchason?)

Examination

Let me feel your pulse.

Déjeme tomarle el pulso.

I am going to take your blood pressure now.

Le voy a tomar la presión ahora.

Respiratory

Vocabulary

Chest

El pecho

Lungs

Los pulmones

History

Do you smoke?

¿Fuma usted?

How many packs a day?

¿Cuántos paquetes al día?

Have you any difficulty in breathing?

¿Tiene dificultad al respirar?

How long have you been coughing?

¿Desde cuándo tiene tos?

Do you cough up phlegm?

¿Al toser, escupe usted flema(s)?

What is the color of your expectorations?

¿Cuándo usted escupe, qué color es?

Do you cough up blood?

¿Al toser, arroja usted sangre?

Do you wheeze?

¿Le silba a usted el pecho?

Examination

Take a deep breath.

Respìre profundo.

Breathe normally.

Respìre normalmente.

Cough.

Tosa.

Cough again.

Tosa otra vez.

Gastrointestinal
Vocabulary

Abdomen	El abdomen
Intestines/bowels	Los intestinos/las entrañas
Liver	El hígado
Nausea	Náusea
Gastric ulcer	La úlcera gástrica
Stomach	El estomago, la panza, la barriga
Stomachache	El dolor de estómago

History

What foods disagree with you?	¿Qué alimentos le caen mal?
Do you get heartburn?	¿Suele tener ardor en el pecho?
Do you have indigestion often?	¿Tiene indigestión con frecuencia?
Are you going to vomit?	¿Va a vomitar (arrojar)?
Do you have blood in your vomit?	¿Tiene usted vómitos con sangre?
Do you have abdominal pain?	¿Tiene dolor en el abdomen?
How are your stools?	¿Cómo son sus defecaciones?
Are they regular?	¿Son regulares?
Have you noticed their color?	¿Se ha fijado en el color?
Are you constipated?	¿Está estreñido?
Do you have diarrhea?	¿Tiene diarrea?

Genitourinary
Vocabulary

Genitals	Los genitals
Kidney	El riñón

Penis	El pene, el miembro
Urine	La orina

History

Have you any difficulty urinating?	¿Tiene dificultad en orinar?
Do you urinate involuntarily?	¿Orina sin querer?
Do you have a urethral discharge?	¿Tiene descho de la uretra?
Do you have burning with urination?	¿Tiene ardor al orinar?

Musculoskeletal

Vocabulary

Ankle	El tobillo
Arm	El brazo
Back	La espalda
Bones	Los huesos
Elbow	El codo
Finger	El dedo
Foot	El pie
Fracture	La fractura
Hand	La mano
Hip	La cadera
Knee	La rodilla
Leg	La pierna
Muscles	Los músculos
Rib	La costilla
Shoulder	El hombro
Thigh	El muslo

History

Did you fall and how did you fall?	¿Se cayó, y cómo se cayó?
How did this happen?	¿Cómo sucedío esto?
How long ago?	¿Cuánto tiempo hace?

Examination

Raise your arm.	Levante el brazo.
Raise it more.	Más alto.
Now the other.	Ahora el otro.
Stand up and walk.	Parese y camine.
Straighten your leg.	Enderece la pierna.
Bend your knee.	Doble la rodilla.
Push	Empuje
Pull	Jale
Up	Arriba
Down	Abajo
In/out	Adentro/afuera
Rest	Descanse
Kneel	Arrodíllese

Neurologic

Vocabulary

Brain	El cerebro
Dizziness	El vértigo, el mareo
Epilepsy	La epilepsia
Fainting spell	El desmayo
Unconscious	La insensibilidad (inconsiente)

History

Have you ever had a head injury?	¿Ha tenido alguna vez daño a la cabeza?
Do you have convulsions?	¿Tiene convulsiones?
Do you have tingling sensations?	¿Tiene hormigueos?
Do you have numbness in your hands, arms, or feet?	¿Siente entumecidos las manos, los brazos, o los pies?
Have you ever lost consciousness?	¿Perdió alguna vez el sentido? (inconsiente)

| For how long? | ¿Por cuánto tiempo? |
| How often does this happen? | ¿Con qué frecuencia ocurre esto? |

Examination

Squeeze my hand.	Apriete mi mano.
Can you not do it better than that?	¿No puede hacerlo más fuerte?
Turn on your left/right side.	Voltéese al lado izquierdo/al lado derecho.
Roll over and sit up over the edge of the bed.	Voltéese y siéntese sobre el borde del la cama.
Stand up slowly. Put your weight only on your right/left foot.	Párese despacio. Ponga peso sólo en el pie derecho/izquierdo.
Take a step to the side.	Dé un paso al lado.
Turn to your left/right.	Doble a la izquierda/derecha.
Is this hot or cold?	¿Está frío o caliente esto?
Am I sticking you with the point or the head of the pin?	¿Le estoy pinchando con la cabeza del alfiler?

Endocrine and Reproductive

Vocabulary

| Uterus | El útero, la matríz |
| Vagina | La vagina |

History

| Have you had any problems with your thyroid? | ¿Ha tenido alguna vez problemas con tiroides? |
| Have you noticed any significant weight gain or loss? | ¿Ha notado pérdida o aumento de peso? |

What is your usual weight?	¿Cuál es su peso usual?
How is your appetite?	¿Qué tal su apetito?

Women

How old were you when your periods started?	¿Cuántos años tenía cuando tuvo la primera regla?
How many days between periods?	¿Cuántos días entre las reglas?
When was your last menstrual period?	¿Cuándo fue su última regla?
Have you ever been pregnant?	¿Ha estado embarazada?
How many children do you have?	¿Cuántos hijos tiene?
When was your last Pap smear?	¿Cuándo fue su última prueba de Papanicolado?
Would you like information on birth control methods?	¿Quiere usted información sobre los métodos del control de la natalidad?
Do you have a vaginal discharge?	¿Tiene descho vaginales?

Index

Page numbers followed by "f" indicate figures, "t" indicate tables, and "b" indicate boxes.

LOOK-ALIKE AND SOUND-ALIKE MEDICATIONS

A Common Cause for Medication Errors

Accolate	Accupril
	Aclovate
Accupril	Accutane
	Monopril
acetohexamide	acetazolamide
Allegra	Viagra
Alora	Aldara
alprazolam	lorazepam
Amikin	Amicar
Ansaid	Asacol
Anusol	Aquasol A
	Aquasol E
Aricept	Ascriptin
Asacol	Os-Cal
asparaginase	pegaspargase
Bumex	Buprenex
	Permax
Cardene	Cardizem
Carafate	Cafergot
carvedilol	carteolol
cefazolin	cefprozil
Cefol	Cefzil
Cefotan	Ceftin
Celebrex	Cerebyx
codeine	Cardene
	Lodine
cyclobenzaprine	cyproheptadine
cyclophosphamide	cyclosporine
Cytosar-U	Cytovene
Cytotec	Cytoxan
Dalmane	Dialume
Darvon	Diovan
Demerol	Desyrel
Denavir	indinavir
diazepam	lorazepam